THE DETOX MANUAL

Also by Suzannah Olivier

. . . .

What Should I Feed My Baby?

The Breast Cancer Prevention and Recovery Diet

The Stress Protection Plan

Also by Suzannah Olivier in the *You Are What You Eat* series

. . . .

Banish Bloating

Maximising Energy

Natural Hormone Balance

Perfect Pregnancy

Allergy Solutions

Suzannah Olivier

THE DETOX
MANUAL

POCKET
B O O K S

First published in Great Britain by Pocket Books, 2001
An imprint of Simon & Schuster UK Ltd
A Viacom Company

10 9 8 7 6 5 4 3 2 1

Simon & Schuster UK Ltd
Africa House
64-78 Kingsway
London WC2B 6AH

Simon & Schuster Australia
Sydney

A CIP catalogue record for this book is available from the British Library

ISBN 0-671-03782-X

The information in this book is designed to make you feel energetic and
healthy. If following a detoxification programme has the opposite effect, you
must stop the programme and check with your doctor or health care provider.
This book includes information about fasting, gall bladder flushes and colon
cleansing. Before embarking on any of these, you must check with your doctor
or health care provider that there are no contra-indications to you following
such programmes.

None of this information is appropriate for pregnant or breast-feeding women,
nor is it appropriate for children.

Herbs and other nutritional supplements are best taken on the advice of a
suitably qualified health professional.

If in doubt about any health issue, always consult your doctor.

Typeset in 12 on 14pt Perpetua with Gill Sans display
Design and page make-up by Peter Ward
Printed and bound in Great Britain by Omnia Books Limited, Glasgow

This book is dedicated to Marjorie, who knows how many 'units' makes a meal in a restaurant . . .

Contents

PART ONE

INTRODUCTION

1   Internal Cleansing   **3**
Drugs or Detox? **3** How Do You Know if You Might
Need to Detox? **4** What Does Detoxification
Involve? **6** How Will You Feel After a Detox? **6**
A Challenge **7** Old Idea, New Approach **8**

2   An Unsavoury Soup   **13**
What is a Toxin? **13** Toxins We Consume **14** Toxins
Produced in the Body **16** Heavy Metals **17**
Pollution **18**

PART TWO

YOUR DETOXIFICATION SYSTEMS

3   Love Your Liver   **23**
The Detoxification Process **26** Damage Limitation **31**
Overburdened **33** Possible Signs and Symptoms of
Reduced Detoxification Capability **35** Sulphur
Compounds **36** Tests for Toxicity **38** Major Diseases
of the Liver **40**

4   Good Housekeeping   **42**
The Intestines **43** Food Sensitivities **44** Sluggish
Digestion **48** Bowel Bacteria **49** Fibre for
Detoxification **49** Skin and Lymph **52** Sweat it Out **54**
Kidneys **56** Cellular Detoxification **57** Fat Cells and
Cellulite **59** Lungs **62**

PART THREE

TIME FOR ACTION

5   **Help Your Liver**   69
6   **Three Plans**   72
    The Three-day Intensive Detox **77** The Ten-day Fix **86**
    The Long-life Plan **94**
7   **Nature's Helping Hand**   106
    Inspirational Juices **109** Supplementing Your Liver **110**
    The Clay Cure **116**
8   **The Purest Drink of All?**   118
    The Solution to Pollution is Dilution **119** Do You Drink
    Enough Water? **120** Quality As Well As Quantity **121**
    Improving Your Water Quality **123** A Cleanser and
    A Healer **124**
9   **Clean Up Your Act**   126
    Home Sick? **126** Avoiding Chemicals **128** Fearsome
    Fats? **132** Alcohol – Liver Enemy No. 1 **134** Coffee
    Cravings **136** The Demon Weed **137** Drugs – Medicinal
    or Otherwise **138** Heavy Metals **140**

PART FOUR

MORE DETOX TOOLS

10 **When Less May be More**   149
    Fasting **149** One-day Juice Fast **152** The Liver
    Flush **153** The Gall Bladder Flush **155** Coffee and
    Camomile Enemas **156** Colonic Irrigation **160**
    Herbal Colon Cleansing **162**
11 **You Can Make a Difference**   163

PART FIVE

APPENDICES

Appendix I – Cleansing Foods   167
Appendix II – Resources   171
Herbal and Nutrient Supplement Suppliers 171
To Find a Nutritional Therapist 173 For Colonic
Health 174 Biochemical Testing 174 Organic Food
Sources 175 Water Distiller Suppliers 175 Suppliers
of Juicers and Other Equipment 175 Suppliers of
Additive-free Personal Care and Household
Products 176 Books 177 Useful Websites 177

Part One

INTRODUCTION

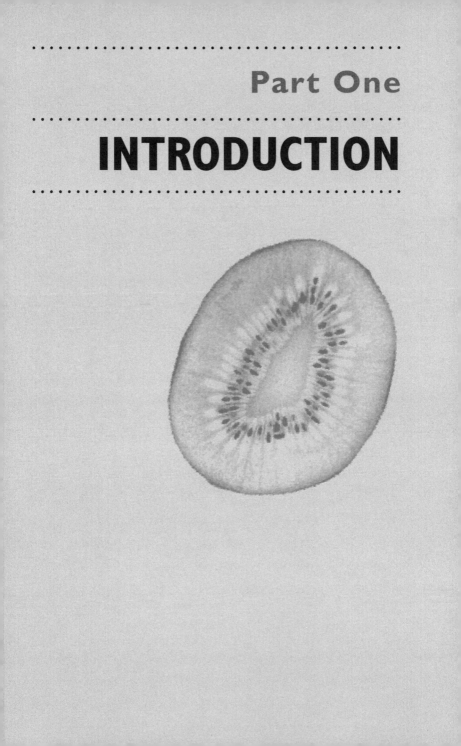

CHAPTER ONE

Internal Cleansing

Just think about how much time you spend on your daily ablutions: you bathe or shower several times a week, clean your teeth twice daily, shampoo and condition your hair two or three times a week, you may even regularly have a massage or sauna. As a society, we worry about body odours, adding scent to our baths and applying it to our skin, and a problem with personal hygiene is soon commented upon at work or at home. Yet despite our obsession with outer cleanliness most people give little thought to their inner cleanliness. Every day debris accumulates in cells, in blood, in the liver, in the lungs and in the colon. Fatigue, sluggish metabolism, lacklustre skin, dull hair and tired eyes are all signs that our bodies are being overloaded with toxins. Cleansing our bodies internally can have significant impact on our appearance. Inner health is reflected in a glowing skin, shining hair and bright eyes.

DRUGS OR DETOX?

Many of those who are drawn to the idea of detoxification are people who have been dealing with a health problem for some time. The majority of these are what I call the 'vertically ill'. The horizontally ill are already being looked after by their doctors, but the vertically ill just put up with a plethora of complaints which plague them from time to time – headaches, aches and pains, low energy, poor skin. These people, and you may be one of them, pick up on the subject of detoxification because they realise that they do not just 'have to live with' their problem, but they may not realise that these uneases (as opposed to diseases) are warning signs.

It is far better to seek the underlying cause of a health problem, rather than to suppress the symptoms with medication. Using painkillers for a headache or bad back is analogous to dealing with the flashing oil light on your car dashboard by unscrewing the bulb or smashing it with a hammer rather than by renewing the oil. The pain in your back is there to tell you not to push your luck and lift heavy objects. The headache is telling you that something is not working properly – for instance, blood vessels constricting in the brain, a food allergy or a tense muscle causing a vertebra to press on a nerve. Use the painkiller judiciously, as a temporary crutch, while you work out the underlying cause, but don't make the mistake of relying on it to mask the symptoms for ever. If you do, the causes are likely to build up and lead to greater ill health later on.

Many cases of ill health, or instances of just feeling 'below par', are linked to an excess of toxicity. Toxins circulate in the blood, are stored in body tissues, affect all areas of the body, including the brain, and lodge in joints. These toxins can contribute to a wide variety of health complaints. If the body is given the chance to throw off this debris it can make a remarkable restoration to full health.

HOW DO YOU KNOW IF YOU MIGHT NEED TO DETOX?

Signs of toxicity are diverse and differ from person to person, depending on their make-up. If you are prone to headaches, they may be made more frequent and severe; if you have a tendency for skin eruptions, you may get a main-crop each time you are under the slightest stress. The following are some of the most common symptoms of excess toxicity:

Possible signs and symptoms of excess toxicity

- bad breath
- coated tongue
- frequent fatigue
- headaches
- cellulite
- inability to lose excess weight
- bowel problems
- digestive problems
- allergies
- high cholesterol levels
- blocked arteries
- gall bladder diseases
- skin disorders such as acne or rashes
- brownish spots and skin blemishes (liver spots)

Symptoms usually flare up when you are under stress. If you have had a bad week at work, are not sleeping properly or are having to make some major decision, signs of toxicity can worsen. This is because the stress causes your energy reserves to be channelled away from your body's detoxification mechanisms.

An unhealthy environment can also affect some people. If you find yourself experiencing symptoms such as spaciness, fogginess, tingling or numbness, an inability to concentrate or depression when in particular situation – for example, using the photocopier or computer, or being exposed to a particular perfume or to cleaning materials – there is a strong chance that your detoxification channels are being over-stressed.

Mental symptoms are just as likely as physical symptoms. The brain is not capable of disarming many toxins and is heavily dependent on the liver to do so. This means that if the liver is not working properly it can lead to a wide variety of mental symptoms, including drowsiness, memory loss, an inability to focus, 'woolly-brain syndrome', and a heightened response to alcohol and other substances.

WHAT DOES DETOXIFICATION INVOLVE?

Detoxification is a two-step process:
- You need to reduce your exposure to toxins in your food, drink and environment to a minimum, by substituting different products and food preparation methods for existing ones.
- You need to give your body the tools it needs to eliminate the toxins it has stored in the past, in order for cells and organs to be able to function at their peak, to repair themselves and to produce energy efficiently.

The tools for encouraging this process include:
- increasing certain foods and drinks in the diet that encourage the process of handling and eliminating toxins
- including certain herbs and nutrients in your regime to speed up the process
- following a 'quick-fix' detox programme that includes a modified fast and perhaps lymph massage or using clay preparations
- working on the negative stress in your life to give your body the space and energy it needs to heal, including using relaxation exercises.

HOW WILL YOU FEEL AFTER A DETOX?

The ultimate aim is to feel terrific. How soon, and how terrific, largely depends upon your state of health to start with, and how seriously you apply yourself to your detox. You may already feel reasonably OK, but are looking for a bit more sparkle in your life. Or perhaps you are struggling against some ailment that you want to eliminate, but for which you have not yet found a solution. It is not unusual for some people to feel worse before they feel better (we will look at this in more detail later), but if you apply the principles of detoxification properly, your health and vitality will soon be enhanced.

You should become bright eyed, clear-headed and energetic. You may also find that you experience dramatic improvements in problems that have plagued you for years, such as a distended tummy, intestinal gas, headaches, skin problems such as eczema and acne, and respiratory ailments such as asthma. In the long term, if you stick to your detoxification programme, and ideally make the principles part of your normal life, you can find that chronic problems, such as cellulite, IBS (irritable bowel syndrome) and migraines can improve beyond recognition or even be resolved.

A CHALLENGE

Recently, in one of the major consumer magazines, an article appeared called 'Detox: Behind The Hype'. According to this, there is no proof or factual basis behind the concept of detoxification. But the one vital ingredient that was missing from the article was an interview with anyone who had actually undergone a detox.

I have seen the results with many clients who sought to enjoy full health. In some case they had been experiencing a period of malaise, or even full blown illness. More often they were feeling generally OK, but believed something was missing. In my experience there is no doubt that most people who follow a detox programme benefit hugely. Within days, bodies that seemed weighed down with the accumulated debris of daily life, feel lighter and cleaner. Mental acuity is sharpened, energy is restored and aches and pains, feelings of heaviness and clogged body tissues are eliminated.

There is only one way to tell if a detox will work for you, and that is to give it a go. I challenge the sceptics to follow an appropriate detox plan seriously, and to discover what many people before them have found, that it can make an enormous difference to how they feel.

A detox can take several forms. The most popular is to embark upon a 'spring clean'. A weekend detox conducted at regular intervals, usually at the beginning of each season, is an effective way of giving your body a chance to throw off accumulated debris and to enhance equilibrium. In truth, however, many of us need to do more than this, and need to make changes both to our diet and to the environment in which we live to reduce our overall toxic load in the long term. This approach will help to improve your immediate health, will probably help you to recover from any health crises that you are experiencing, and may even help you to avoid some of the major degenerative diseases in the future. Detoxing is a voyage of discovery as you peel away the layers of health problems, eating habits and the environment in which you find yourself living, and can be an enlightening experience. This book will take you through the various options, and give you a choice of eating plans to realise your aims. Enjoy the process of achieving vitality and inner health.

OLD IDEA, NEW APPROACH

Why is it that so many people are drawn to the idea of detoxing? What is it that we are looking for? The vogue for detoxification is probably linked to the growing awareness of the impact that our environment can have upon our health. Perhaps it is also a way in which people feel that they can regain control of their physical being in the face of a seemingly unavoidable onslaught of chemicals in our food, water and homes.

The idea of body detoxification is not a new one, and is common to many societies across the globe. Different approaches have been used: fasting is a practice in many cultures and religions, and enemas and colonics are a feature of many health cures. Some eastern mystics advocate drinking one's own urine as a means of cleansing body tissues, and Himalayan yogis have been known to swallow lengths of cloth and pass them through their system. Despite there being a resurgence of interest in the ancient practice of detoxification, you will be pleased to hear that the means do not need to be quite so dramatic!

Detoxification is the means by which the body rids itself of any unwanted chemicals. These chemicals can be the waste products of your own body processes and of the bacteria and other foreign bodies, such as germs, which inhabit your intestines. They can also enter your body from the air you breath, the food and water you consume, and substances that are absorbed through your skin. In fact, in the industrialised world, it is virtually impossible to breathe or eat without taking in toxic chemicals. Nearly every molecule the body deals with, including those which are naturally produced, needs to be disarmed and eliminated once it has served its purpose. Typical examples of this process include dealing with the ammonia which is left over after proteins have been used, disarming hormones which have served their purpose, and getting rid of dead cells that have been removed by the immune system. This process is an expensive one, physically speaking, using up a large part of the energy the body expends on metabolism.

The liver and kidneys are the main organs invloved in eliminating toxins. The skin and bowels are also major organs of elimination. Keeping these in peak condition allows us to feel clear-headed and energetic.

The issue of toxins – and therefore detoxification – centres on two important themes:

● **The type and strength of toxins to which we are exposed** Extreme examples of this occur when workers in particular jobs, such as agriculture, chemical plants or dry cleaners, are adversely affected, sometimes seriously, by their work environment – the victims of Gulf War syndrome are still trying to prove their case. More mundane examples of exposure to strong toxins are people who drink or smoke heavily and who pay the price with their health.

● **The individual's ability to deal with those toxins** We all have differing capacities for detoxification. The detoxification capabilities between different people may vary by as much as five fold, because of their genetic make-up. Two people in the same car may be exposed to the same rush hour smog, one may feel fine while the other may develop itchy eyes, an irritated throat, runny nose and headache.

It is likely that the person who exhibits signs of excess toxicity, such as a sluggish metabolism, a feeling of permanent tiredness, adverse food reactions, or multiple chemical sensitivities, is not as capable of handling the load as the next person. There are a number of reasons why this may be so, and we will look at these later in the book.

In 1927 Johanna Brandt wrote a book called *The Grape Cure*, which detailed her return to health after following a mono-food fast using grapes. In the book she talks about The Seven Doctors of Nature, which she listed in the following order: Fasting, Air, Water, Sunlight, Exercise, Food and Mind. Her ideas have stood the test of time and remain as relevant today as when she devised them. Let's look briefly at each of these 'Doctors of Nature', but in an order that I prefer, with an up-to-date view point of each.

1   **AIR** Without breath we are not alive – taking breath is the first thing we do when we are born and the last thing we do on this earth. Learning to breathe deeply to fill the lower part of our lungs allows proper circulation of oxygen to the tissues. Air quality is important, and while there is little that we can do to avoid the pollution of, say, inner cities, there is much that we can do to improve our body's resistance to the pollution, and to improve the air quality in our homes. We will cover these points later.

2   **WATER** After air, water is the second most vital nutrient, without which we cannot live. Looking after the quality of your water, and drinking plenty of it, is one of the most important health-giving steps you can take. A whole chapter in this book is devoted to this subject.

3   **SUNLIGHT** Along with both other animals and the plant kingdom, we respond to sunlight. Although we have managed to punch a hole in the ozone layer, and it is obvious that extended exposure to intense sunlight can lead to skin damage, regular exposure to gentle sunlight, sufficient to manufacture vitamin D in our skins, is a vital element of a health programme. Getting out of doors daily, however, especially in the winter months, is something many people no longer do, as we live and work cloistered in buildings.

4   **MIND** An important part of any detox programme is to balance our mental energies and to focus on our goals. In addition to detoxing our bodies, we can also get rid of our mental clutter. This usually involves creating a calm environment with a minimum of distractions, which enables us to channel our energies and resolve whatever is giving us cause for worry. When you achieve this, then you can truly

say that you have been detoxed! Destructive emotions, such as hate, fear, self-pity and resentment create their own toxicity by affecting hormone balance, digestion and blood flow.

5   **EXERCISE** We are made to move. To remain static, behind a desk or in front of the TV, for hours and even days on end, only serves to seize up our joints and weaken our muscles. Moving does not necessarily mean a strenuous workout, it can be an invigorating walk, getting on with physical tasks that you have been putting off, or merely enjoying life – just make sure you move around regularly. Massage is another way of getting the body 'moving', and while it is not a substitute for exercise, it is a potent tool for encouraging the body to throw off toxins.

6   **FOOD** The quality of the food we eat is the main focus of this book. You wouldn't put substandard fuel in your brand-new Rolls-Royce and expect it to perform, so why put substandard or the wrong food for your body chemistry into your mouth? In addition to food, there are a number of herbs that have been shown over the millennia to be effective at encouraging restoration of health by supporting the major organs of detoxification. Concentrated nutrients can also provide this support. We will look at these later.

7   **FASTING** A modified fast (in which certain foods are allowed, rather than just a water fast) is one of the quickest ways of allowing your body to repair itself. Even if you do not manage to fast as often as you would like, you can still fast from particular substances. If you have never gone for a month without coffee, then now is your opportunity to do so, and to see how you reap the benefits. Fasting is something that your body understands, you just need to make your mind understand it as well.

An Unsavoury Soup

Soup recipe: 6 stewed slugs, 75 g minced rat's entrails, 2 desiccated eyeballs, a sprinkling of compost, all mixed in with 250 ml pond water. Doesn't sound very attractive does it? In fact, no more palatable than this: 2 measures of ethanol, a sprinkling of formaldehyde, a pinch of benzene, a soupçon of methylxanthines and a dash of dioxins. Yet the ingredients of the second soup recipe are consumed by large numbers of people every day, without a second thought.

WHAT IS A TOXIN?

What exactly is a toxin? It can be defined as any substance which is detrimental to cell functioning, and therefore to the optimal health of the body. During normal functioning, our bodies process an enormous number of such substances. They may be ones which we would normally expect to cope with, such as carbon dioxide in the air, or the debris that our bodies produce as a by-product of digestion and cell repair or as a result of fighting bacteria or other organisms. But increasingly the toxic substances are coming from foreign chemicals which have been introduced into our environment in recent decades. In our grandparents' day there were far fewer chemical and synthetic pollutants. Of course, some people were exposed to serious health hazards which are not countenanced today, such as asbestos and coal dust, but the majority of people in earlier times did not have to deal with the cocktail of thousands of chemicals to which we are now exposed. Over the past fifty years, humans have had to adjust to an astounding number of chemicals, which place a huge burden on the liver and on other detoxification systems. The broad categories of sources of toxins to which we are exposed include:

● toxins we consume
● toxins produced in the body
● heavy metals
● pollution

TOXINS WE CONSUME

Natural toxins in foods: Even the person who eats an unprocessed, organic diet needs to have an efficient detoxification capability because many of the foods which we eat come with a supply of substances which are toxic and need to be neutralised and eliminated. When we eat familiar foods, such as potatoes, celery, parsnips and mushrooms, we eat toxic compounds that are intrinsic to the food. Common examples of these natural toxins are glycoalkaloids in the green part of potatoes, lectins in red kidney beans and algae-induced toxins in shellfish. It is also common to find toxic moulds and fungi on our foods, and mould will grow on bread in a warm environment in only a couple of days. Mycotoxins such as patulin in mouldy or damaged apples, and aflatoxins in peanuts, milk, grains and figs are other examples.

Provided we eat a varied diet, these do not present a problem, but there are examples of problems caused by overconsumption. In the 1960s, a whole community in India was struck down with poisoning by toxic lathyrogens due to overconsumption of chickpeas. There have also been several deaths attributed to eating potatoes that have been exposed to the light and allowed to grow green shoots. Proper food preparation, such as cooking kidney beans thoroughly, eliminates many of the plant toxins, but if they are present in large quantities in incorrectly prepared food, or if a person's detoxification capability is below par, the consequences can be serious.

Chemicals and additives in foods: These days we are exposed to a wide variety of added compounds in our food. There are in the region of 3,000 additives in daily use in commercial food production, including preservatives, stabilisers, artificial colourings and flavourings, and gases used to artificially ripen fruit. A huge number of chemicals used in farming, such as pesticides, fungicides, insecticides and artificial fertilisers find their way on to our plates. Testing on the safety of these residues tends to be done on individual compounds, but the long-term effects of the whole chemical soup are only just beginning to be looked at and are possibly quite alarming. Around 50 per cent of the antibiotics in circulation are used for meat production as growth enhancers, and these appear in the meat and milk products we consume. Not only do these antibiotics add to our chemical load, they are also suspected of contributing significantly to the problem of bacteria superbugs which are now becoming resistant to treatment in humans. Another potent source of chemicals is our water supply – around 800 regularly find their way into drinking water.

Non-food foods: This may seem to be a contradiction, but it is deliberate. There are a number of substances we ingest – I hesitate to call them foods – that are comparatively recent additions to our diet. Coffee and sugar were both introduced in the last few centuries, while more recent examples include colas and other novelty drinks. And while alcohol has been used by most cultures around the world for thousands of years, it also comes into this category. The common factor with all of them is that they are not necessary for our bodies to function – and if consumed in any quantity, they are actually detrimental, are significantly addictive, and are major sources of toxins. They will be covered in more detail later in the book.

Drugs: As a society, we depend upon a plethora of drugs. The most ubiquitous are nicotine and alcohol, but recreational drugs, such as marijuana, are also a feature of many people's lives these days. In addition, we take for granted a wide range of over-the-counter drugs, which, if taken to excess, can induce organ toxicity sufficient to be hospitalised. And, of course, there is also prescribed medication. At the turn of the century, GPs only had a dozen or so drugs at their disposal, but they now have more than 4,000 to chose from, and if you read the list of side effects caused by the majority of them, you will find that a toxic effect on one organ or another is exceptionally common. It has got to be better, if possible, to treat the cause of an illness rather than suppress it with multiple-medication. (You must not, of course, abandon any prescribed medication without first consulting your doctor.)

TOXINS PRODUCED IN THE BODY

Bacteria and yeast, which are resident in the gut, produce a number of compounds, some of which are toxic. If there is insufficient fibre in the diet, or if bowel movements are not regular, there is ample opportunity for these toxins to be absorbed across the gut wall and into the bloodstream. Gut-derived toxins have been implicated in a number of diseases, including all the inflammatory digestive diseases (gastritis, colitis, Crohn's disease, coeliac disease, excessive gut permeability), liver disease, thyroid disease, diabetes and immune problems, including allergies, arthritis and asthma, to name but a few.

Toxins are also produced in the body on a daily basis as a result of protein digestion. Proteins are mainly found in meat, poultry, fish, dairy produce, eggs, nuts, seeds, soya, beans and pulses. When proteins are used by the body they produce residues such as urea and ammonia. These residues are mainly eliminated by the kidneys, which need to be supported by ensuring that adequate water intake is maintained. We need proteins for most body functions, and to repair and build tissues, but problems can arise when an excess of proteins are eaten, as is typical on a Western diet.

HEAVY METALS

Many metals, such as gold and silver, are stable and do not usually cause the human body a problem. But some of the metals to which we are exposed are toxic and, because they are easily absorbed, can cause quite a bit of damage. Such metals, because of their chemical composition, are called 'heavy metals'. If you think for a moment of the Mad Hatter in the book *Alice in Wonderland* you will know of the toxic effects of mercury on the brain (mercury was used in the hat-making process until the early part of the 20th century). The other main toxic metals to which we are exposed are lead, cadmium, arsenic and aluminium. Their absorption can take place over a long period of time, from a number of sources, resulting in a slow build up. This slow build up can lead to a gradual accumulation of adverse symptoms, which are often mistakenly attributed to other causes. Common sources of heavy metals are industrial processes, petrol, pesticide sprays, cooking utensils, domestic water pipes, cigarette smoke, dental fillings, old paint work (flaking off or chewed by children), anti-perspirants and antacid medication. Elimination of these heavy metals from your body can be encouraged and this is covered in more detail in **Clean Up Your Act**, page 126.

POLLUTION

It is impossible to avoid pollutants in today's world, even if you go to the far reaches of the earth. Pollutants are carried around the world in the most alarming way — significant levels have been found in the ice caps at the two Poles, and in the milk of breast-feeding Inuit women. The chemical industry has quadrupled in size in the last 30 years and accounts for 10 per cent of total world trade. Over 100,000 different chemicals are registered for commercial use in Europe alone, 60,000 of which are in regular use, yet little is known about toxicity or the long-term safety of the vast majority of these. Of particular concern is the compounded effect of these various chemicals — the effect of chemicals has been studied in isolation, but what effect they may have together is completely unresearched.

But what we can do is to protect ourselves as far as possible from the effects of pollution? Practically speaking, we can reduce our exposure to chemicals significantly by being selective about our buying habits and food preparation methods. We can also encourage our bodies to eliminate a certain amount of the accumulated toxins.

It has recently been estimated that we are exposed to around 300–400 volatile organic (carbon-based) chemicals in our homes on a daily basis. This is made much worse by the fact that our houses are better insulated than in earlier days. We have centrally heated and draught excluded our homes, to the point where these chemicals cannot escape and as a result recirculate and build up. We are exposed to a number of chemicals from fire retardant fabrics, mattresses, stain resistant carpets, dry-cleaning fluids, cleaning materials, insecticides, fungicides, fumes from our gas boilers, pressed-wood and fibreboard furniture, insulation materials, and even from our washing machine cycles. For instance, chlorination of our water leads to airborne toxic chemicals, such as toluene, ethylbenzene, cyclohexane and acetone, being liberated. These are vented into the kitchen, and the rest of the house, when we use dishwashers.

We are even being accosted by EMFs (electromagnetic fields), which are another form of pollution. There is sufficient concern about EMFs for the World Health Organisation to be funding major studies on their effects. These EMFs come from computers, TVs, mobile phones, fridges, electric clock/radios and electric blankets. If you feel groggy when you get up in the morning, despite sleeping a reasonable number of hours and being in generally good health, you may want to consider dispensing with the electric clock/radio by your head, the electric blanket and even, in these automated days, the electrically cantilevered bed. (You might also be reacting to substances in your duvet, pillows or mattresses.)

Out of doors it is not much better, with traffic levels expected to rise by one-third nationally in the UK over the next 20 years, and to quadruple in some rural areas. Inner city pollution is dropping, but levels nationally are rising steeply.

This may seem like an overwhelming and impossible situation, but it is not difficult to find health-friendly substitutes to products you already use once you are aware of the possible downsides of living in an overly polluted home. Not everyone needs to address these issues as a matter of urgency, and usually addressing diet is sufficient to restore health. However, if you find that you are struggling with long-term health problems that will not resolve themselves, focusing on the environment in which you live can bring relief.

Part Two

YOUR

DETOXIFICATION

SYSTEMS

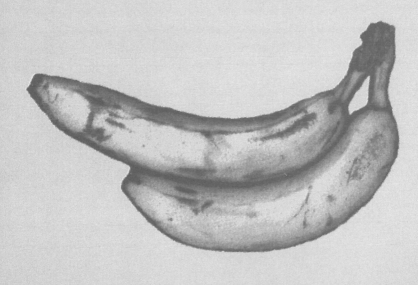

CHAPTER THREE

Love Your Liver

The liver is an astounding organ, which you must learn to love if you want to maintain your body's ability to clear out toxins at peak performance. It is our main organ of detoxification, and can be thought of as a cleansing filter for your bloodstream, clearing out unwanted substances and micro-organisms by neutralising and disposing of them.

Apart from the skin, the liver is the largest organ in the human body – it weighs around 1.3kg and is about the size of a football. It is responsible for more than 40 essential functions, and in addition is a chemical factory making many different enzymes which perform more than 500 different tasks. The liver also has the amazing ability to regenerate itself, as long as it is not too damaged.

The liver, however, is a little appreciated organ, which does most of its work in silence – it doesn't beat (like the heart), it doesn't relax or contract (as do your muscles), it doesn't rumble (as your digestive system may do), we are not aware of its processes (as we are with our kidneys or our bowels), and it has to go really badly wrong before we start to think about its health. Because the liver can more or less still function with up to 80 per cent deterioration, symptoms of its ill health can be vague and they may not be identified with the liver until the damage is severe.

Activities of the liver include

Making cholesterol Cholesterol is both made and processed
by the liver. If you need to make more cholesterol for
making sex and stress hormones, it can do so, and if you
have too much damaging cholesterol it is designed to
redress the balance – if it is given the chance!

Making bile More than a litre of bile is made daily to emulsify
(break up) fats from the diet. Some bile is excreted from
the bowels and carries with it toxins for disposal.

Keeping energy levels constant The liver produces quick
energy in emergency situations, or in between meals, by
releasing glucose (sugar) into the blood. It also produces
long-term energy, as needed, by converting food energy
into the metabolic energy and nutrients which cells need
for them to function. Excess blood glucose is also turned
into fat when too much sugar and refined carbohydrates,
such as white bread, white rice or sugary cakes and biscuits, are eaten.

Stoking the furnace The liver is the powerhouse that gen-
erates the heat needed to keep your body warm. If it is
working too hard you can feel hot and bothered, or if it is
sluggish you may feel your energy levels are well below
par.

Storing nutrients Certain vitamins are unable to be
absorbed, or used, unless they are carried in fats. The liver
is a storehouse of these fat soluble vitamins – vitamins A,
D, E and K. It also stores vitamin B12 and the minerals
iron and copper, along with smaller amounts of most other
minerals.

Manufacturing proteins Proteins are made up of chains of
amino acids linked together in different combinations.
There are only eight essential amino acids, from which all

the others can be made. This involves a process called transamination, where amino acids are reshuffled to make different proteins, which takes place in the liver.

Activation of hormones Hormones such as oestrogen, thyroxine, aldosterone and the active form of vitamin D are processed through the liver, making the health of this organ crucial for hormone balance.

Detoxification The liver's job in dealing with toxins is to make them harmless, so that they can be eliminated via our urine, faeces, sweat or breath. This process involves two clear stages – Phase 1 and Phase 2. There is also another process which limits damage to the liver during the course of these two phases. The importance of these stages is explained in the next section.

Signs and symptoms that your liver may be out of sorts can include: digestive disturbances, a metallic taste in the mouth, headaches, drowsiness after meals, loss of appetite, an inability to tolerate fatty meals, low energy levels, 'dinginess' in the whites of the eyes, perpetual dark circles under the eyes, jaundice, pale stools or pain on the right side of the upper abdomen.

As one of the liver's jobs is dealing with fats and cholesterol, liver health is an important consideration in all forms of fatty degeneration diseases – or diseases where fatty materials are found in places where they are not meant to be, such as blocked arteries and obesity. Several problems can be linked to the poor use of the fat-soluble vitamins (vitamins A, D, E and K) by a liver that is working below par or insufficient bile production.

THE DETOXIFICATION PROCESS

To understand the process of detoxification it is worth exploring a little more deeply the way in which the liver is involved. If you are not particularly technically minded you can probably skip this section (though it is not too taxing!) and go straight to **Good Housekeeping** on page 42. However, if you have any long-term health complaint which is not resolving itself, or if you want to know more about the workings of this marvellous organ, read on.

Filtering the blood

One of the main jobs of the liver is to filter the blood and 'sieve' out toxins and other compounds. The blood is loaded up with live bacteria, toxic products from dead bacteria and substances the immune system has disarmed. Each and every minute, around 2 litres of blood is filtered and during this process around 99 per cent of the bacteria and toxins should be removed before the blood goes back into general circulation again. Liver damage will compromise the effectiveness of the filtration system leading to health problems.

The gall bladder and bile

Another means by which the liver is involved in detoxification is by off-loading toxins in the bile. Bile is made in the liver and is drip-fed into the gall bladder. This sac is where the bile is concentrated, making it more effective at beginning the process of digesting fats by emulsifying them. Around a litre of bile is made daily. The bile ends up in the bowels, and a large amount of it is then reabsorbed for re-use. That which remains in the bowels, however, is the means by which a number of fat-soluble toxins are eliminated in the faeces. A diet high in fibre is essential for this process to work properly, as it allows the toxins to be bound properly into the faeces. If this does not happen they can be reabsorbed into the bloodstream, instead of being eliminated.

If the excretion of bile is inhibited, toxins are forced to stay in the liver for longer than they ought to. There are several reasons why this might happen, such as obstruction of the bile duct by gallstones and reduced bile flow within the liver. It is estimated that around 20 per cent of people over the age of 40 have gallstones (10 per cent of the general population), and women are three times more prone to them than men. Gallstones are mainly composed of cholesterol, and the link between diet and gallstones centres on a high-fat and low fibre diet, which is typical of that eaten in the West. People with gallstones are also more likely to have a diet that is low in vitamin C and to have low blood levels of this vitamin. Bile flow interruption can be linked to gallstones, high levels of toxins from bowel bacteria, an overactive thyroid or excess thyroid medication, pregnancy, oral contraceptives, anabolic steroids, liver disease such as hepatitis, hereditary diseases such as Gilbert's syndrome, and a number of drugs. The most common cause of impaired bile flow, however, is alcohol, and in sensitive individuals, or in alcoholics, the effect can be significant.

Gall bladders are commonly removed in 'spare part' surgery as a result of gallstones. It is often suggested that the gall bladder is not needed as its job is only to concentrate the bile, and if it is removed this simply means that the bile will drip into the digestive tract to do its job anyway. In reality, gall bladder removal can result in a significant reduction in digestive capability and can, in turn, lead to later health problems because of inefficient fat digestion. If you are threatened with gall bladder surgery, you may want to turn to page 155 where a 'gall-bladder flush' is described (though it is only suitable for small sized gallstones). It is not pleasant, but it is effective and may be better than surgery. If you have already had your gall bladder removed, the most effective way of compensating for its function is to sprinkle a couple of tablespoons of lecithin daily on your food. Lecithin is described in more detail on page 110 in Supplementing Your Liver (Nature's Helping Hand).

P450 Detoxification

The other means by which the liver deals with toxins is by the P450 detoxification enzyme system, which is broken down into Phase 1 and Phase 2.

Phase 1

The first stage is known as Phase 1. The substances which trigger this phase include caffeine, alcohol, proteins in excess of the body's needs, charcoal barbecued meat, steroid hormones such as the female and male sex hormones and the stress hormones, and man-made chemicals such as cigarette smoke, exhaust fumes, paint fumes, drugs, organophosphates (from farming chemicals) and dioxins (from processing plastics, industrial wastes and other materials).

Phase 1 does not actually get rid of most toxins, just packages them ready for elimination in a process which makes the molecules more 'sticky' (so they attach themselves to other molecules) and more soluble (which aids excretion). There are a series of liver enzymes which are a part of Phase 1, which belong to a family called the P450 enzymes. The more toxins you are exposed to, the harder the P450 enzymes have to work. You may be surprised to find that many of the end-products of Phase 1 are even more toxic than the original substances, and the significance of this is discussed below.

For the P450 enzymes to work properly there needs to be a

plentiful supply of a wide number of nutrients, including the
B-vitamins, glutathione, healthy fats (including those called
phospholipids), and a large dose of antioxidants. All of these are
provided by a healthy diet and are discussed in **Supplementing
Your Liver (Nature's Helping Hand)**, page 110.

Some substances that trigger P450 enzymes

acetate	exhaust fumes
alcohol	high protein diets
barbiturates	organophosphates
caffeine	paint fumes
carbon tetrachloride	saturated fats
charcoal grilled meats	steroid hormones
dioxins	sulphonamides

Phase 2

Phase 2 is the stage that disarms the toxic products that result
from Phase 1, and allows the body to eliminate them.

In Phase 2 the end-products of Phase 1 have substances
'stuck' to them to render them harmless and easily excreted
(this is called conjugation). By this process the toxic 'sticky'
compound is made larger and less toxic. For instance,
glutathione is stuck on to certain toxins, and this is how we
detoxify the drug paracetamol. If a person overdoses on paracetamol, he or she is given N-acetyle cysteine (which is quickly
converted into glutathione) to mop up the highly damaging
toxins that result from Phase 1 and which can induce fatal liver
damage.

Sulphur is another vital compound which is used for this
process and it is used by the body to neutralise the toxic compounds which come from the Phase 1 processing of compounds
such as steroid hormones (for example HRT and the Pill, as well

as natural hormones, and paracetamol). Sulphur is concentrated in foods with a strong smell, such as garlic, onions and eggs (in fact it is the sulphur which gives them this characteristic). Other foods which are good sources of sulphur include cottage cheese, red peppers, asparagus, cabbage, Brussels sprouts, broccoli, cauliflower, mustard and horseradish. Meat is another good source of sulphur, but is best eaten in moderate quantities.

Along with these two detoxification routes (glutathione and sulphation) there are two other key detoxification routes – glucoronidation and glycine. Together these four pathways are responsible for dealing with substances such as alcohol, antibiotics, aspirin, paracetamol, toxic metals, chemicals from cigarettes, tranquillisers and hormones. Some compounds found in foods are particularly useful for improving their performance, or 'upregulating' them. Some of these foods are the cruciferous vegetables (broccoli, cauliflower, cabbage, Brussels sprouts), foods which contain limonene (citrus peel, dill weed oil and caraway seed oil), sulphur containing foods (garlic, onion, eggs, cottage cheese), fish oils, cystein containing foods (wheatgerm, oats, yoghurt, cottage cheese, turkey) and benzoic acid containing foods (berries, prunes, cloves, cinnamon, anise). Certain vitamins and minerals (B-vitamins, magnesium, selenium and zinc) are also critical for these pathways to operate properly.

The detoxification steps all work together, which means that if one is overloaded there is a reasonable capacity to process the toxins by another pathway. However, if there is serious overload, or if there are not enough nutrients (vitamins and minerals) to support all the options, the system cannot cope as well and efficiency is compromised. What can also happen is that one of the alternative pathways converts chemicals into chloral hydrate (the consituent of a 'Mickey Finn' or 'knock-out drops'). Some people who have been exposed to certain chemicals which overload their ability to detoxify – chemicals such as glues, dry cleaning fluids, paint or new carpets – behave in the same way as if they had been given a Mickey Finn.

Along the way there can also be 'bottlenecks' in the system. At each stage, certain nutrients are needed for the action to take place. If these nutrients are lacking the bottleneck is worsened, rather like a car slowing to a crawl in the narrowed lane of a busy road which is undergoing repair works. Around one in three people is, according to official statistics, deficient in at least one essential nutrient.

The nutrients and compounds which are used for conjugation in Phase 2, and which act to remove offending toxins from the body, are, once used, lost for ever. This means that the process uses up energy and nutrients on a daily basis, and we need to replenish stocks regularly in order to maintain the efficiency of the system.

DAMAGE LIMITATION

As already mentioned, at the end of Phase 1, and before Phase 2, some substances are even more dangerous or toxic than in their original state. For instance, many are oxidised, creating harmful free radicals (see explanation below), which can damage the liver cells. In order to minimise this we need a good supply of antioxidant enzymes and nutrients. These include vitamins A, C and E, flavonoids such as quercitin and limonene, minerals such as selenium and zinc, as well as the potent antioxidant glutathione, which is needed by the liver in large quantities. Fruit and vegetables in our diet are the main sources of these valuable antioxidants.

Many of the pollutants we encounter increase our exposure to free radicals. Free radicals are unstable molecules that are missing an electron. This is an unnatural state for them – nature likes balance – and so they seek to stabilise themselves by

attracting an electron from another source. If that source happens to be our body tissues, damage is caused to our cells. They
usually pair up with our cell enzymes and cell membranes and
so can be extremely disruptive to the work of the liver.

Research suggests that free radical damage is involved in
premature ageing, and is implicated in at least 50 of our most
prevalent diseases, including heart disease and cancer. Sources of
these free radicals from our environment include the sun, radiation, exhaust smoke, factory emissions and cigarettes. Free radicals are also derived from our diet, and are made worse by
foods that speed up metabolism, such as sugar and alcohol.
Damaged fats, including vegetable fats used in food processing
and cooking, are also responsible for free radical damage.

Free radicals are produced as a result of natural body
processes such as breathing and digesting food, so they are
something that our bodies are normally meant to be able to deal
with. Unfortunately, however, we have overloaded our bodies
with excess sources of free radicals by exposing ourselves to
pollution and to adverse dietary factors.

Sources of free radical damage
- Natural body processes, such as metabolism, breathing,
  digestion and liver detoxification.
- Dietary factors, such as sugar, alcohol and an excess of
  processed grains (such as white bread and white rice). Also
  hydrogenated fats found in margarines and commercially
  prepared foods (such as crisps, pies, biscuits and roasted
  nuts), as well as in rancid and overheated vegetable fats.
- Environmental factors such as the sun, car exhaust, factory
  emissions, cigarette smoke and radiation.

Protection from free radical damage

- Natural body antioxidant enzymes produced by a healthy liver.
- Dietary sources of antioxidants, such as fruit and vegetables and their juices, but also teas, herbs and olive oil.
- Avoidance of sources of free radicals (such as cigarette smoke, radiation, sugar, alcohol or drugs, etc).

OVERBURDENED

Problems commonly arise when Phases 1 and 2 are out of synch with each other. If Phase 1 is working at full pelt in an attempt to package up excess amounts of toxic compounds for the next stage, but Phase 2 is not working efficiently, possibly because it has long since been pushed to the limit of its effectiveness, or because the compounds needed for Phase 2 conjugation are not available from the diet, the result can be a large number of even more toxic compounds doing the rounds. The implications of this can be quite serious for some people.

One in ten people take painkillers on a daily basis, yet a significant number of people find that if, for instance, they take headache medication, it will actually make their headache worse and not better. The reason for this is likely to be that they are unable to detoxify the by-products of the medication, which then contributes to their overall toxic load, and leads to more headaches. Instead of suppressing symptoms with drugs and making the situation worse, what they probably need to be doing is following a detox programme.

Recent research has also confirmed that those who use paracetamol on a daily basis double their risk of developing asthma, and those who take it once a week have an 80 per cent increase in risk (asthmatics are unable to take aspirin as it can trigger serious attacks). The researchers suspect that the reason for this is that the paracetamol reduces levels of glutathione, one of the important detoxifying substances, leaving the body more susceptible to pollutants.

Genetically, there is no doubt that some people have a lesser ability to detoxify compounds compared to others, and this can have serious consequences. For instance, women with naturally reduced levels of the enzyme N-acetyl transferase seem to have a higher risk of breast cancer if they smoke. The lung cancer risk for smokers is increased in the case of people who have reduced capability of another detoxification enzyme, glutathione transferase. These people are simply unable to cope with the extra toxic burden of smoking. Of course, by avoiding smoking, you avoid overburdening these enzyme systems.

To summarise, the main process of detoxification looks like this

Inhaled, ingested or absorbed
foreign chemicals, or by-products
of natural body processes

↓

Phase 1 detoxification ⟶ Some products are excreted in urine

↓

Some more toxic compounds
formed, which can damage liver
tissue. Antioxidants protect from
much potential damage.

↓

Phase 2 detoxification ⟶ Excreted in urine or in bile in the gut

Any of these stages can be blocked or damaged by
- vitamin or mineral deficiency
- protein deficiency or overload
- eating too many of the wrong types of fats
- foreign chemicals that the body is unable to detoxify
- an excess of newly formed breakdown products from Phase I
- detoxification enzymes interfered with by heavy metals
- detoxification pathways overloaded by everyday chemicals
- genetic deficiency (i.e. lack of particular enzymes)

POSSIBLE SIGNS AND SYMPTOMS OF REDUCED DETOXIFICATION CAPABILITY

Apart from the general signs of possible toxic overload (see page 4) there are some interesting signs and symptoms that can give clues as to the state of your liver and its ability to detoxify. Phase 1 may be working below par if there is even mild caffeine intolerance or if perfumes and other chemicals make you feel unwell. On the other hand, if you are able to tolerate large amounts of caffeine and, say, are able to drink two cups of coffee late at night without it affecting your ability to sleep, then it is possible that you have an overactive Phase 1. Yellowing whites of the eye (not due to hepatitis) can indicate a sub-functioning Phase 2, and toxemia during pregnancy (pre-eclampsia and eclampsia) is also an indication of reduced activity of Phase 2.

Chinese restaurant syndrome (caused by the additive MSG), which results in symptoms such as headaches, nausea, weakness, sweating and flushing, may indicate that there are low levels of a substance called glutamate decarboxylate, which prevents the MSG being processed properly. Some people are helped by taking 100–150 mg of vitamin B6, which restores this function (B6 is always best taken alongside a B-complex which enables all the B-vitamins to work together).

The sulphation phase of detoxification may be operating below par if you have an adverse reaction to foods containing sulphur compounds (sulphur dioxide, sodium sulphite or disulphate, metabisulphite), such as dried fruit, instant mashed potato, wines, processed meats, beers and ciders. It was common for vulnerable people to experience bad asthma reactions when eating at salad bars in restaurants until the practice of using sulphur containing preservatives was stopped. Other signs that the sulphation phase may not be working properly are if garlic makes you feel sick, or if eating asparagus makes your urine smell very strongly.

Researchers at Breakspear Hospital in Hertfordshire, which specialises in environmental medicine, have found that many patients with multiple chemical sensitivities (i.e. having unpleasant reactions to small amounts of chemicals or pollutants) do not have an efficient sulphoxidation process. In addition, people who suffer from migraines, and who react to chocolate, cheese and oranges, are suspected of having a problem with making sulphates. As a result, such people are unable to process the tyranine in cheese or the octopamine in oranges (both naturally occurring substances) using sulphates.

If testing (see below) shows that sulphate capability is reduced, sulphate levels can be raised using two crystals of Glauber's salts dissolved in hot water or soup daily. (Glauber's salts are an inexpensive, old-fashioned remedy for short-term constipation, and are available from pharmacies. They consist of sodium sulphate.)

SULPHUR COMPOUNDS

You may have noticed that I have talked about sulphur as a compound found naturally in foods, which is needed to encourage the sulphoxidation detoxification process in the liver, but I have

also said that sulphur preservatives are problematic. To clarify
the situation:

- Sulphur found naturally in foods as sulphur amino acids
  (protein building blocks) is beneficial – rich sources
  include onions, garlic, leeks, eggs, cottage cheese, ricotta
  cheese, avocado, wheatgerm, meat and wild game.
- Nutrition supplements which include sulphur containing
  amino acids or MSM (methyl sulfonylmethane) may also be
  useful for helping the detoxificaton process. MSM is a sulphur compound which is naturally found in mother's milk
  and in very fresh produce. It is used in the detoxification
  process and in the production of high energy molecules.
  MSM has been used in the treatment of a number of conditions which benefit from detoxification, particularly asthma, arthritis, allergies, hay-fever and lung problems. It
  helps to flush out heavy metals, such as mercury, and has
  also been used to eliminate parasites. Until the 1940s, sulphur was mixed with molasses to make a vile tasting concoction that was used to deworm people, particularly those
  living in rural communities.
- Foods which contain sulphur oxide and sulphur dioxide
  preservatives may present a problem, as it is thought that
  the oxide and dioxide component increases oxygenation
  damage to tissues. It is not usually necessary to avoid these
  compounds, but it may be prudent to limit them, especially if you have health problems such as asthma.
- Foods containing some types of sulphates or sulphites, on
  the other hand, do seem to have health implications. They
  are converted in the liver to harmless sulphates, but,
  before this happens, sensitive people can react allergically
  (particularly asthmatics, but others as well) and they can be
  viewed as another toxin. These compounds are often listed

as sodium bisulphate, sodium metabisulphate or potassium metabisulphate, and are found in dried fruit, dehydrated vegetables, grapes (and grape juice and wine), mushrooms, desiccated coconut, vinegar, peeled potatoes and potato products and other foods. The E numbers to look out for are E221–E227. Confusingly, E220 is a collective term which may mean sulphur dioxide (see point above) or could also mean any other sulphite/sulphate E-numbers in combination.

TESTS FOR TOXICITY

You don't necessarily need to have a test to know if you are carrying an excess toxic load, and it's worth remembering that tests can never be entirely conclusive. By far the best indicator is how you feel before and after a detox programme. However, it may be appropriate for you to talk to a health professional about carrying out tests, particularly if any of the following apply:

● your health has not improved fully after a concerted health programme of several months
● you are diabetic
● you have, or have had, gallstones
● you have a history of heavy alcohol or nicotine use
● you suffer from psoriasis or another severe skin condition
● you have used natural or synthetic steroid hormones for an extended period of time, e.g. anabolic steroids, HRT or oral contraceptives
● you have had frequent exposure to chemicals or drugs, e.g. cleaning solvents, pesticides, antibiotics, diuretics, non-steroidal anti-inflammatory drugs, thyroid hormones, recreational drugs
● you have a history of liver disease.

These are the most useful tests:

Hair mineral analysis

A hair mineral analysis is by far the most useful test to discover if you have an excess of heavy metals. It is simple, non-invasive, and relatively inexpensive. A sample of hair is taken from the 5cm of growth nearest the nape of the neck and a note made if the hair is dyed or permed. It is then sent to a laboratory to be analysed. As heavy metals are excreted from the body into the hair, the sample should give a fairly accurate idea of levels in the body during the previous two to three months. A dietary programme, designed to encourage the elimination of toxic metals, can then be devised and, once it has been followed for six months, the test can be repeated to see how effective it has been. It is important that the test is carried out by a reliable laboratory, a list of which appears in the **Appendix**, page 174, and it should not to be confused with other hair tests advertised in the back pages of health magazines which encourage samples of hair to be sent for analysis by other methods, such as dowsing.

Tests for microbial compounds

Urinary indican test This looks for markers which indicate excessive bacterial putrefaction in the bowels or breakdown of proteins. Urine tests can also look for protein breakdown products, bile pigments and other compounds.
Stool culture This looks for an abnormal microbial concentration and for disease causing organisms.
    Both these tests are best conducted via a nutritionally trained doctor or a trained nutritional therapist.

Detoxification profile

The standard liver function tests carried out by your doctor are only useful at diagnosing if there is a serious clinical problem. By the time you get significant test results you may well be horizontally ill rather than vertically ill. If, however, you have had a liver function test from your doctor which gives results that require monitoring but not immediate medical action, a programme of liver support including, for instance, the herb milk thistle (see page 108), may be beneficial.

A more useful test of liver capacity for most people is the Detoxification Profile. This is capable of picking up lowered liver enzyme function before the situation manifests as a chronic health problem. The test involves taking in a specific amount of caffeine, aspirin and paracetamol. By measuring substances which appear in the urine it is possible to tell whether your liver is able to detoxify these chemicals well enough. It can pinpoint whether Phase 1 and Phase 2 are working in synchronicity with each other, or if there is an imbalance between the two. These tests are best undertaken with the help of a nutritionally trained doctor, or a qualified nutrition consultant, who can interpret them. To find a consultant see **Resources**, page 173.

MAJOR DISEASES OF THE LIVER

Major diseases of the liver include fatty degeneration, where damage, often caused by alcohol or drugs, leads to fatty deposits in the liver, reducing its ability to function. This happens, to an extent, in anyone who abuses their liver, but is only considered medically significant when the degeneration is severe, possibly resulting in an enlarged liver. Hepatitis is an inflammation of the liver and comes in several forms: A, B, C and delta. It can be caused by viral or parasitic infection, or by alcohol, drugs or toxins, as well as by blood transfusions. Cirrhosis of the liver is a laying down of fibrous tissue in the liver, which interferes with its functioning and is most evident in heavy alcohol drinkers. Continental countries, such as France, are renowned for having vastly less heart disease than the UK or US. This is largely attributed to their intake of red wine, which is a rich source of protective antioxidants, yet they also have one of the highest death rates from sclerotic livers – a case of pick your poison! There are also hereditary liver problems, such as Gilbert's syndrome, the main sign of which is constantly elevated levels of bilirubin in blood samples, as the liver is not effective at breaking down red blood cells. It is generally considered that nothing can be done about this problem, and that there is a greater risk in such people of jaundice. However, a natural approach of detoxifying the liver with diet and other naturopathic means, as well as using herbs such as milk thistle have been shown to be effective at normalising bilirubin levels. Cholestasis is an interruption in the flow of bile from the liver into the digestive tract, and it can be caused by hepatitis, drug or alcohol use, liver cancer or even by pregnancy.

Good Housekeeping

Of course, your liver does not go it alone completely, and the body's detoxification processes are complex, involving a number of different organs. For a complete picture of how your body handles toxins, it is helpful to look at the wider picture. The other parts of the body which are involved in handling toxins are as follows:

Intestines
- Fat soluble toxins are eliminated via the bile which, in turn, is excreted through the faeces.
- Toxins from bowel bacteria are disarmed by the mucus membranes of the bowels.

Skin and lymph
- Fat soluble toxins such as pesticides, and some heavy metals such as lead are excreted in sweat.
- You can think of the lymph system as your body's waste collection system. Lymph carries white blood cells around the body, and through the lymph nodes, to deal with unwanted foreign infections, cell debris and other toxins.

Kidneys
- Our kidneys filter around 150–200 litres of blood daily! Toxins which have been made water soluble by the liver are excreted through the urine. The kidneys also keep our blood alkaline by filtering out dissolved acid wastes.

Individual cells

- In addition to the major organs of detoxification, the process also needs to go on efficiently in most cells in the body. To encourage efficient cellular detoxification we need to eat a diet which is principally 'alkaline' in nature (see below).

Fat cells and cellulite

- Toxins which are unable to be eliminated are stored either in the liver or in fat cells. In some people, women especially, this may make cellulite worse.

Lungs

- The lungs filter out toxic substances from the air we breath, remove toxins from the blood and eliminate carbon dioxide.

THE INTESTINES

Most people are aware that we get rid of waste matter through our bowels, but wrongly assume that a large amount of it is toxic waste. While the intestines are an important contributor to the processing of toxins, the bulk of our stools is actually indigestible plant matter, and around one-half of the weight of our stools is made up of bacteria.

Intestinal health contributes to the elimination of toxins in three principal ways:

- Many irritants come from the foods we eat, and we can be sensitive to them. How the digestive tract responds to these irritants affects the levels of toxins in the gut, which then affects the liver.
- The efficiency with which bile is eliminated, and therefore

the toxins that the bile carries, is greatly influenced by the amount of fibre in the diet.

● The balance of the bacteria in the bowels between 'friendly' and 'unfriendly' bacteria, affects whether or not they contribute to our toxic 'load' by secreting chemicals to which we are sensitive. The balance of bacteria is also influenced by the amount of fibre in the diet.

FOOD SENSITIVITIES

Food allergies and sensitivities are a common phenomenon and contribute to the whole problem of excess toxins. If your body is having an adverse reaction to a particular food or drink, it is inevitably being overtaxed. Food sensitivities are often caused by a knock-on effect that begins with the digestive system. The digestive tract is irritated by foods that do not agree with it, which triggers the immune system to attack the 'foe' and causes the detoxification systems, particularly the liver, to go into action. In a classic chicken-and-egg situation, liver problems can contribute to the build up of such sensitivities, which in turn can contribute to compromised liver health. Signs that you may be sensitive to a food, or group of foods, include symptoms such as bloating, wind, diarrhoea, constipation, weight gain, headaches, migraines, mucus problems, asthma, acne, eczema, psoriasis, arthritis or even a tendency towards depression or anxiety.

If you suspect that you have an adverse reaction to any particular food, it is wise to avoid it. By far the worst sensitivity problems arise from wheat and cow's milk products, and from the stimulants sugar, alcohol and coffee. Both wheat (and other grain) products and cow's milk are staples of the Western diet and, as a result, we are susceptible to eating too many of them. You may want to experiment with avoiding foods to which you believe you are reacting for a trial period of at least two weeks.

If you find that you are sensitive to them, you will know that your body has been having to deal with stress caused by the residues from their digestion. One of the most obvious indications that you are eating a food which is likely to affect you adversely is if you are in any way attached, or addicted, to it. This is because the food to which you are sensitive stimulates the stress hormones, and these then play havoc with your brain chemicals leading you to feel you cannot live without whatever it is. The best way out of this situation is to:

1   Identify which foods may be causing you harm and over-taxing your detoxification systems. In addition to the foods and drinks already mentioned, the other common foods that cause problems include yeast, corn, potatoes, oranges/citrus fruit, rye, soya, peanuts, eggs, shellfish, tomatoes and chocolate.
2   Organise yourself to buy a good number of other food options which will allow you to eat without missing the foods you are avoiding.
3   Make a meal plan which is realistic and allows you to enjoy your food. Ensure that you have enough time for meal preparation, or that you know where you can buy fast, easy meals that fit into your eating plan. Read the **Three Plans** on page 72 for some ideas on how to get started, and adapt them to suit your tastes and needs.
4   Set a definite date by which you will start your programme, and keep a note of any changes in symptoms that you have – good or bad. This will allow you to become more in tune with your body's reactions to foods.

The following is a checklist of alternatives to the two main foods that are likely to be causing problems.

Alternatives to wheat Wheat is found principally in bread, pasta, pies, cakes, biscuits, pastry, breaded products and cous-cous. It is also found in packaged sauces, meat products such as sausages, malted products and products using modified starch. One of the problems with wheat is that it finds itself in just about any processed food, as it is a cheap filler ingredient. If you find that you need to eliminate wheat, eat products made from other grains. You can experiment with:

- **rye:** used for rye crackers, which are available in many varieties, 100 per cent rye bread, which has a slightly sour, but pleasing, taste, pumpernickel bread and rye bread.
- **oats:** available as oatcakes, porridge oats and oat flake top-pings for sweet or savoury dishes.
- **rice:** can be used as a basis for curries or in salads, in a dish on its own, such as brown rice risotto, and also comes as rice cakes and rice noodles.
- **corn:** available as sweetcorn, polenta or maize flour (which can be used to make delicious cornbread and wheat-free cakes), cornflour, popcorn, corn pasta, burri-tos, tortillas and corn chips (but check to ensure no wheat has been included in the ingredients list).
- **buckwheat:** buckwheat noodles are the basis of many Japanese dishes and are delicious in soups. Blinis (Russian pancakes made with buckwheat flour) can be topped either with apple sauce, sliced strawberries or nut butters, or something savoury such as fish paté or chopped herrings. They freeze well when interleaved with greaseproof paper and can be warmed up individually as an instant alternative to bread.
- **millet:** available as flakes, which can be used to make por-ridge; as grain, which can be cooked like rice; and as puffs, which can be eaten for breakfast.

- **quinoa:** the grain cooks like rice, and quinoa flakes and puffs are available as breakfast cereals.
- **barley:** the grain is a good substitute for rice. It is also available as flour.
- **other:** filling starchy foods are usually well tolerated if grains such as wheat cause a problem, and can provide a bulky basis to a meal instead of using bread or pasta. Use root vegetables such as potatoes, sweet potatoes and yams, and sago or tapioca for desserts. You can also experiment with flours made from chickpeas or lentils which, along with products such as poppadums made from these flours, are available from Eastern food shops.

Sticking to a new eating plan is most difficult when you are under time pressure, so it is best to plan ahead and stock up. Instead of a sandwich at lunchtime, have a baked potato, some thick soup or a salad. You can have rye crackers, oatcakes or rice cakes instead of bread, either adding a variety of toppings or eating them plain to accompany meals. Instead of wheat based pasta, try some of the numerous other types of pasta made from different grains which are available from health food shops.

Alternatives to cow's milk products If you are snacking on cheese or milky drinks all the time, there is a chance that you may be sensitive to dairy produce, especially if you have symptoms that include mucus in the respiratory tract, upper respiratory tract infections or asthma.

There are so many dairy alternatives now available that you need never feel deprived. Soya products are excellent these days and include milk, yoghurts and cheeses. You can also find rice, oat and coconut milks, and oat fibre based yoghurts. You may find that despite being sensitive to cow's milk, you can still enjoy modest amounts of sheep's, goat's or buffalo milk products. So cheeses such as goat's cheese, halumi, feta and mozzarella can remain on the menu. The one cow's milk cheese that appears to be OK for most people who are sensitive to dairy, is Parmesan. This is because the proteins are broken down in the ripening process, making them more easily assimilated, and most of the lactose is removed. Live yoghurt is often well tolerated for the same reasons.

SLUGGISH DIGESTION

As a society we tend to be constipated, and only one person in three evacuates their bowels daily. To eliminate toxins from the bowels efficiently, we need to have healthy bowel movements daily. On a typical Western diet we produce between 80–160 g of faeces daily, whereas vegetarians produce, on average, around 225 g daily. African villagers, on the other hand, who eat a traditional, highly fibre-rich, diet top the charts with a magnificent 470 g daily.

We should get the 'urge' to go naturally, and when we do we should not override this need and wait until later. There should also be no straining involved. Any parent will know that babies fill their nappies soon after they are given a feed, as a meal automatically stimulates the urge to eliminate the bowels. As children and adults we learn to ignore this automatic reflex, and in time this can lead to a spastic bowel and sluggish elimination. Sluggish digestion is a contributor to the problem of build up of toxicity because bile, and the toxins it carries for elimination, have more time to be reabsorbed. For proper elimination it is vital to get enough fibre. Frequently, people will use a variety of means to help them go to the bathroom, including a morning cup of coffee, cigarette or, even worse, laxatives. These do nothing to help and simply stress the digestive system further, leading to an even more sluggish bowel. The bowel is a muscle which needs to be exercised, and fibre in the diet is the way to exercise it.

BOWEL BACTERIA

If you have not been going to the lavatory properly for a long time, and have been eating foods which do not agree with you, it is a fair bet that the balance of bacteria in your bowels will favour bacteria which are 'unfriendly'. You can acquire even more unfriendly bowel bacteria by the simple method of eating more sugary foods such as pastries, biscuits, sweets and chocolates, drinking a little too much alcohol, drinking sodas, and taking antibiotics, steroid drugs or the Pill. This is a shame, because the 'friendly' bacteria that they displace in our bowels have important detoxification functions – functions with long names such as hydrolysis, dehydroxilation, decarboxylation, dehalogenation and aromatisation. The unfriendly bacteria also produce huge numbers of chemicals which are toxic to our systems and which irritate the gut wall and overtax the liver. In addition, they produce an enzyme in our bowels called beta-glucoronidase. This enzyme has the unfortunate habit of liberating toxins which are about to be eliminated in faeces and freeing them up for reabsorption.

For the full run down on digestive health, see *Banish Bloating*, another title in this series of books.

FIBRE FOR DETOXIFICATION

Refined foods, such as white bread, which have been stripped of their fibre, have been popular throughout the centuries with those who could afford them (they were expensive until industrial scale refining became possible in the 20th century). Dissenters, however, warned of associated health problems. In

1583, the Puritan pamphleteer Philip Stubbs commented: 'Doe we not see the poore man that eateth browne bread healthfuller, stronger and living longer than the other that fare daintelie every day?'

Unrefined foods are the source of fibre in our diet. The most important function of fibre is to regulate bowel movements. Fibre reduces the absorption of toxic substances created by the activity of gut bacteria. In particular, the water-soluble fibres found in fruit, pectin, oat bran, psyllium and linseeds are efficient at binding with toxins and promoting their excretion via the bowels. By reducing the absorption of toxins into the bloodstream, the 'load' placed on the immune system and the liver's detoxification systems is reduced and a considerable saving of energy is made.

There are two main types of fibre, insoluble and soluble. Insoluble fibres are mainly found in wheat and vegetables. They increase fecal bulk and speed up the passage of faeces through the intestines. Soluble fibres are mainly found in fruits, beans, oats and barley. They bulk faeces but also delay the absorption of glucose into the bloodstream and lower blood cholesterol levels.

Fibre is a 'regulator' and is necessary to help avoid constipation, but also to regulate diarrhoea. So the same solution is needed for both conditions. Fibre is also the most important factor in the long term for balancing the bowel bacteria. If you are wary of fibre because in the past it has made your condition worse, this means that you need to go more slowly when introducing it into your diet. Initially, perhaps, eat more fruit, which has been peeled. Then start to eat the peel on the fruit. Then introduce some of the fibres mentioned below at a slow pace. It is also worth considering the type of fibre you have used in the past. Often people experience problems because they are sensitive to the source of fibre, and this is particularly the case with wheat products, particularly high bran cereals.

The most useful fibres for detoxifying

- **vegetables and fruit** In addition to being valuable sources of antioxidants and compounds which support the liver enzyme systems, these foods should also make up the bulk of our diet to contribute soluble fibre. Particularly rich sources of fibre include prunes, pears, raspberries, figs, peas, beans and lentils. It is best to not peel your fruit or vegetables (where appropriate) to get the most fibre from them, however do wash them properly, whether organic or not, and ideally choose organic produce.

- **pectin** This is a fibrous gel, rich sources of which are apples, pears and bananas. It is particularly useful for absorbing toxins, especially heavy metals such as aluminium. Apple pectin is readily available from health food shops.

- **oat bran** Using oat bran instead of its more familiar cousin, wheat bran, can help to keep fibre levels up without irritating the gut wall. Oat fibre is proven to lower cholesterol levels and to stabilise blood sugar levels. It is also highly successful at mopping up toxins.

- **psyllium** This is the ground up husk of the plantain seed and it is soft, cooling, lubricating and mucus clearing. It also absorbs toxins. Psyllium husks are fantastically useful for regulating bowel movements if there is the slightest sign of constipation or diarrhoea, as it forms a gelatinous mass which keeps faeces soft, bulky and hydrated. In this way it also stimulates the reflex contractions of the bowel walls. Add it to fruit juice and drink it before it thickens too much. A teaspoon or two of psyllium taken daily by the entire population would probably halve the rate of digestive diseases, as well as diabetes and cardiovascular diseases. It has the same cholesterol lowering effect as oats,

but you only need 10–12 g instead of 3–4 generous serv-
ings of porridge! It has no known side effects except that
you poop more!

● **linseeds** These are best ground up to release their rich
load of essential fats. These fats are terrific for reducing
inflammatory problems. The seeds are rich in glycosides,
which prevent muscle spasms of the colon, and lignans,
which help to protect against breast cancer.

*Fibres have their most potent effect in combination, giving the advan-
tages of the different types*

SKIN AND LYMPH

Skin and lymph have been grouped together because external
treatments, which might seem to be mainly of benefit to the
skin, will also help to mobilise lymph and encourage detoxification.

Skin
. . . .

The skin is the body's largest organ which, if spread out, would
cover around 1.5 square metres (20 square feet). Skin helps to
regulate temperature and body moisture content, and in a normal day we lose around half a litre of sweat, or much more if we
are physically active or if it is a hot day. The skin will also act as
a back-up route of elimination for other organs if they are not
able to work properly. If, for instance, the bowels are not working effectively, it is common for this to make spots, acne and
other skin problems worse as toxins are off-loaded via the skin.
The ability to lose compounds in the sweat is apparent when you
consider how the smell of something pungent such as garlic or
curry spices quickly makes its way into the sweat.

Lymph

Lymph is a clear fluid which circulates in the lymph system and is responsible for bathing all the cells and keeping them cleansed. It carries waste from the cells of the body to the elimination organs. Major lymph glands are the appendix, spleen, thymus and tonsils. We have many smaller lymph glands dispersed throughout the body, which range in size from that of a tiny pea to that of a kidney bean. The lymph system is a major part of the immune system, and toxins and other organisms, such as bacteria, are filtered through and disarmed in the lymph glands. There is around twice the mileage of lymph channels as there are blood vessels in the body, and the lymph which circulates in these channels needs to be kept free-flowing.

One of the features which distinguishes the lymph system from the arterial system is that there is no pump, such as the heart. The way that lymph is moved around the body is by valves, which keep the lymph flowing in a particular direction, and by contractions of the major muscles exerting a pressure on the system. This means that being active, movement and taking exercise is important if the lymph system is to do its job properly. If lymph is stagnant cleansing of the tissues does not work effectively. The best way of keeping the lymph clear and free-flowing is to drink plenty of water (around 2 litres daily), to eat a diet rich in watery foods, such as fruits and vegetables, and to keep the amount of saturated fats from animal produce in your diet to a minimum as they slow lymph down.

The most dramatic sign of lymph which is pooling and not circulating properly is oedema, or swelling of tissues. This is usually worse around the legs, ankles and feet, but can also affect areas such as the upper arms when lymph glands have been damaged, for instance by surgery.

. . . .

SWEAT IT OUT

There are a number of methods which can help to encourage the
lymph to flow and speed along the passage of toxins out of the
lymph, and to encourage them to be eliminated in sweat.

● **exercise** will improve all aspects of health, contributing
(depending on the type of exercise) to cardiovascular
health, suppleness, strength and mental calmness. One of
its more important but lesser known benefits is to keep
lymph flowing through the channels by the pressure of
muscles against the vessels. Brisk walking for at least 20
minutes a day will improve circulation and help your body
to eliminate toxins through the skin. Aerobic exercise,
which makes you sweat, is even more helpful at encouraging the movement of harmful chemicals and heavy metals
out of the body in the sweat. It can also serve to get rid of
pent up emotions, the stress of which can contribute to
feelings of toxicity.

● **dry skin brushing** is a tried and tested way of encouraging
healthy lymph flow and speeding up the elimination of toxins. It involves using a natural bristle body brush (synthetic
bristles damage skin), of the type you can buy from a good
pharmacy, and using it on dry skin in long sweeping
strokes. Use a dry brush on dry skin, and always travel up
the body from the toes, or fingers, up towards the heart.
The whole process should take about three minutes.
Include the soles of your feet, the palms of your hands and
your neck and head, though be cautious about your face.
Use firm strokes, but do not rub yourself raw. After you
have done this you can have your bath or shower. Skin
brushing obviously dislodges dead skin, opens up pores and
improves circulation, but it also enhances the movement of
lymph through the lymph channels and encourages the

elimination of toxins from the skin. Do not brush over any areas of broken skin. In the long term, the combined effect of dry skin brushing along with alternating hot and cold showers has been shown to increase resistance to infections, and in the short term they give a wonderful feeling of rejuvenation.

● **anything which encourages improved circulation** will enhance the loss of toxins through the skin. Turning the shower from warm to cool or cold is refreshing and not as difficult as it may sound. The effect of alternating temperatures stimulates the immune system to the extent that it has been suggested by some doctors that the number of cases of colds and other upper respiratory problems could be halved by doing this on a regular basis. The herb ginkgo biloba can also help to improve circulation, and has been useful in cases of poor circulation, which can lead to memory impairment, cold extremities and even sexual dysfunction.

● **health spa treatments** such as saunas and body wraps will all help to increase elimination of toxins through the skin. It has actually been found that drug detoxification programmes which use regular saunas to encourage sweating have significant merits over those that don't as the drugs are eliminated through the skin.

● **tongue scraping,** strange though it may sound, is another way of encouraging the elimination of toxins via the skin. It involves using an inexpensive, simple, flat edged tool to literally scrape the coating off the tongue to reduce the number of bacteria in the mouth. The mouth is a warm, moist environment which is ideal for bacteria to proliferate and the rough structure of the tongue provides a large surface area for unwanted debris and micro-organisms to accumulate. This simple method helps to reduce the overall load. Gum disease, sore throats, sinus problems and gastro-intestinal conditions can all be diminished by tongue scraping. Tongue scraping is, surprisingly, more effective than tongue brushing with a toothbrush, and is recommended by the British Dental Association.

KIDNEYS

The entire volume of our blood is filtered through the kidneys about 20 times each hour. We lose around 1–2 litres of urine daily, and the volume is affected by a number of factors, including liquid intake, blood pressure, the concentration of solutes in the urine, diet, temperature and whether or not diuretics are being used.

We need to replace this liquid by drinking water, but also by eating a diet which is high in watery foods such as fruits and vegetables. These foods are also high in the mineral potassium, which benefits water balance in the body. High levels of salt in the diet, and of toxic materials to filter out, will severely increase the workload of the kidneys.

The kidneys keep the blood alkaline by filtering out dissolved acid wastes (alkalinity is the opposite end of the scale to acidity). You can help to keep your kidneys in peak working order by drinking plenty of pure water. To support the correct alkaline/acid balance further, drink 250 ml of alkalising fresh juice daily. The most useful of the alkalising juices are watermelon, celery, cucumber, buckwheat sprouts and sunflower sprouts, though virtually any fruit or vegetable will be highly beneficial (see Inspirational Juices, page 109).

If your urine is cloudy or smells stronger than is usual, drink larger amounts of pure water to flush through and cleanse your kidneys (unless you have kidney disease in which case consult your doctor).

To keep our kidneys in good working order certain herbal teas are of great benefit. Goldenrod (*solidago*) is a marvellous remedy, the leaves and flowers of which can be made into a tea that is drunk up to three times daily (it also available in ready-made preparations). Other herbs which act as urinary antiseptics include angelica root, bearberry, celery seed, cranberry, juniper, saw palmetto and yarrow. Do not self-prescribe herbs if you have kidney disease or kidney stones, but see a qualified herbalist, in addition to your doctor. Also, do not take herbs if you are pregnant or breast feeding.

CELLULAR DETOXIFICATION

So far we have been talking about detoxification in terms of the health of organs, yet disarming and disposal of toxins also happens in most cells in the body. Each cell is like a mini-factory with a nucleus acting as the command centre. Within the cells there are minute 'organelles' or cell-organs which have specific roles. Some of these are responsible for packaging and eliminating wastes. For these activities to work effectively the right conditions need to be in place. Cells are principally alkaline. There are certain areas of the body which are meant to be acidic, namely the stomach, parts of the intestines, the surface of the skin, the saliva and the urine, but principally we are designed to be alkaline entities. As a result, we are designed to eat a diet which is rich in alkaline enhancing foods.

Interestingly, the foods which enhance alkalinity are not always those which are alkaline in their basic state. For instance, a raw lemon is highly acidic, but when it is digested it has an alkaline effect on the body, as do all fruits and vegetables. The foods which are alkaline in their effect are those which promote the health of other areas of the detoxification system, such as the liver, the bowels, the skin and the kidneys, so eating an 'alkaline forming' diet is compatible with what we have already discussed.

If the body is exposed to 'acid forming' foods (mainly proteins found in meat, fish, dairy produce, grains and beans), it needs to turn the resulting acid residues into alkalines. Certain organs, such as the liver and the pancreas, can only function if they are kept alkaline and blood is kept strictly in the range of 7.35–7.45 pH, which is ideal for carrying oxygen. If blood is unable to be kept at this level a condition called acidosis develops which, if it becomes extreme, is dangerous, leading to coma and even death. Obviously the body does not allow this to happen unless the system has really broken down, so it channels a lot of its energy reserves into alkalising the acid residues of certain types of foods. There are a number of 'buffering' systems which use certain minerals, such as calcium and potassium, to carry out this process within cells. Alkalinity is considered to be 'anabolic' or 'building' of body tissues, while acidity is considered to be 'catabolic' or 'destructive' of body tissues. In the short term, an acid forming diet stresses the cells' detoxification capabilities, making the process that much more difficult and less efficient, and leading to a heavier burden being placed on the liver. One of the more serious long-term consequences of eating a highly acid forming diet for many years is that calcium is leached out of the bones to maintain the status quo in cells, at the expense of bone health. This is one of the most important contributing factors to osteoporosis, a bone disease that affects 1 in 3 women and 1 in 12 men. In such cases the bones end up looking like sponges with holes where the calcium is meant to be, which leads to fractures and broken bones.

Acid forming foods: protein foods such as meat, poultry, game, fish, eggs, milk, cheese, beans, lentils, pulses, grains, nuts and seeds. Sugar.

Alkaline forming foods: all fruits, all vegetables, sprouted
seeds, sprouted nuts, sprouted grains, plus the following
protein exceptions: almonds, brazils, yoghurt and buckwheat (because their mineral make-up allows them to be
metabolised in an alkaline manner).
Neutral: fats.

It is not necessary to cut out all acid forming foods – this is nei-
ther practical nor desirable, as we need sources of good quality
proteins. The trick is to achieve the right balance between the
two food groupings. Ideally, you need to be eating around 70 per
cent of your foods from the alkaline-forming food group and 30
per cent from the acid-forming food group (this equation
ignores fats which are neutral). In practice, this means getting
into the habit of looking at your plate and visually seeing if your
meals achieve this sort of balance. So if you are having a ham
sandwich with bread (grains), ham (protein) and sliced tomato
and lettuce (alkaline vegetables) the balance is more likely to be
70 per cent acid forming and 30 per cent alkaline. On the other
hand, if you have a ham salad with lots of salad vegetables,
avocado, olives and some strips of ham and a sprinkling of
sunflower seeds, then you are achieving the opposite, desirable
balance of 70 per cent alkaline forming foods and 30 per cent
acid forming foods. If a 70/30 balance seems like too much to
achieve initially you might want to at least aim for a 50/50
balance.

FAT CELLS AND CELLULITE

Fat is a major way in which the body stores toxins. If we are
unable to eliminate the toxins, we must find a place to put them
out of harm's way. And fat cells are the ideal place to do this.
Here we store fat soluble toxins such as the by-products of

chemicals which come our way from the household, agricultural and industrial chemicals we ingest, absorb or breathe in. Because of this, it is a good idea, when on a weight loss programme, to lose weight slowly. Not only is this likely to be the best way of keeping weight off, but it also minimises the number of toxins which are released from the fat cells into the body. If they are released too speedily, this places a burden on the liver and can lead to an overload of oxidation damage. Losing around 0.5kg/1lb a week is ideal.

Cellulite may well be a sign of excess toxicity with the toxins stored in the fat cells of the thighs. Cellulite is a common problem for women, particularly on their thighs. Part of the reason why women have cellulite problems is that their fat structure under the skin of their thighs is different to that of men's. This subcutaneous layer of fat is arranged in fat cell chambers with radiating and arching dividing walls of connective tissue (whereas in men it is arranged in a criss-cossing pattern). The 'pinch' test will tell you if you have a cosmetic problem with cellulite. When pinched a 'mattress' pattern appears with pitting and bulging of the skin. If this effect is achieved in men, it is possible that this is a sign of low levels of androgens, the male hormones.

One reason for cellulite may be that, in women, there is a need to keep toxins away from any potentially developing foetus, and so during the reproductive years toxins are stored in the lower body in preference to in the liver. One of the key ways of eliminating cellulite is to lose weight and to do plenty of fat-burning aerobic exercise. However, it is perfectly possible to find slim women with cellulite, and to find large women without cellulite, which suggests that weight loss is not all there is to the equation. Certainly, improving the structure of connective tissue is of great value, but detoxification plays an equally important part in dealing with cellulite. Because toxins stored in fat are a means of long-term storage, it also follows that it can take a significant amount of time to eliminate the problem. Fast weight loss may make the mattress phenomenom more apparent if the strength of the underlying connective tissue cannot keep up. If you are unable to lose weight, take comfort in the fact that detoxifying your body, usually over a significant amount of time – possibly a couple of years – can lead to the elimination of cellulite, even if you do not lose weight.

Vigorous dry skin brushing (see page 54) for 5–10 minutes daily can greatly enhance local detoxification and help to reduce cellulite. In addition to using the long sweeping motions up towards the heart, you can also use circular movements over the affected area. You need to be persistent and to keep detoxification and skin brushing going for several months to achieve an effect. In skin care specialist Liz Earl's book, *Natural Beauty*, she recommends a massage oil that consists of 100 ml grapeseed oil, 1 tsp wheatgerm oil, 10 drops juniper essential oil, and 5 drops each of lemon and fennel essential oils. Applied to the area daily after bathing, using a firm, circular motion, it is, says Liz, effective at helping to break down the dimpled effect on thighs.

There are also some additions to your routine which may help to eliminate cellulite. All are available from good quality health food shops.

lecithin This phospholipid may help to disperse pockets of fat under the skin. Take a tablespoonful twice daily for at least three months.

gotu kola When taken orally three times daily for at least three to six months, gotu kola has been shown to help get rid of cellulite where other treatments have failed. It seems to work by improving connective tissue structure by stimulating the manufacture of cosaminoglycans, and so reducing the formation of hardened connective tissue. In one study of 65 people, who had tried other therapies for three months, good results were experienced by 58 per cent and satisfactory results by 20 per cent.

horse chestnut The key compound in horse chestnut, aescin, has anti-inflammatory and anti-swelling properties and is useful both for lower leg water retention and for treating cellulite. It helps to reduce the size and number of small pores of the small capillaries, making them stronger and less prone to damage, which improves general circulation in the legs. Horse chestnut can be taken as a herb tincture or tablets, or used topically, and is also good for varicose veins.

bladderwrack/kelp This, along with other seaweeds, is high in the mineral iodine and because of this probably helps the thyroid to tune up the metabolic rate. Topical application of bladderwrack has a soothing and softening, as well as a toning, effect on the areas where cellulite tends to accumulate, and is a favourite spa treatment.

It is important to remember, however, whatever treatment you follow, that getting rid of the cellulite won't necessarily be the answer to all your prayers because we all have different genetic shapes and some people inevitably have fatter thighs than others.

LUNGS

Another route by which chemicals get into your body is through your lungs. Within seconds of them hitting the capillaries in your lungs particles are in your bloodstream. It may be an unnerving thought that a part of almost everything around you gets into your system. Everything is continually undergoing breakdown and, as this happens, molecules are released and can be breathed in. This is why you can smell cut melon from several feet away.

There are also less pleasant smells of which this is true! Equally, you don't have to smell something for it to be infiltrating your system – for example deadly carbon monoxide is odourless and undetectable.

For some people, such as those who have asthma or bronchitis, airborne pollutants are no joke. Some particularly unfortunate people even have what is called environmental illness (EI). It is not uncommon, however, for such people to be branded hypochondriacs, despite the fact that there is no doubt that some people are highly sensitive to a number of factors in their environment. If you have respiratory problems, or think that EI might be an issue, you need to look further afield at detoxifying your environment, dealing with moulds (damp places such as kitchens and bathrooms are the worst), flooring, such as carpeting which traps dust and mites, household chemicals and bedding materials. For some suppliers of suitable products see **Resources**, page 176. Your lungs will thank you if you make improvements in your living and working conditions to make them pollution-free environments as far as possible. Keep your home and office well ventilated, and avoid using products which leach chemicals in to your air (see **Clean Up Your act**, page 126). Some people also find that they benefit from using an air ioniser, particularly if they live in an area of high pollution. This is a machine which changes the electrical charge of the air around you to mimic that which is more likely to be found near the sea.

Some foods are particularly beneficial at strengthening the mucous membranes in the lungs and improving lung capacity. Recent research has shown that an apple a day really does keep the doctor away. Researchers looked at fruit and vegetable intake and found that eating just five apples a week made a marked improvement to lung function and capacity. And it was apples rather than other fruits and vegetables that made the difference. When they adjusted for other factors, such as general diet, age, fitness, social class and other fruits and vegetables eaten, it was the apples which stood out. It is thought that this is down to a specific antioxidant which is rich in apples called quercitin. Other sources of quercitin are onions (especially red onions), red wine and tea.

Dark red berries contain proanthocyanidins, antioxidants which are particularly potent at helping to maintain lung health. A serving daily of cherries, blueberries, raspberries, blackberries or other berries can make a significant difference. In the winter-time frozen or canned berries can provide these precious antioxidants (though avoid those canned in sugar or syrup).

As already mentioned, the various types of dairy produce are the foods most likely to be involved in respiratory tract problems and if you suffer from colds, infections and mucus, you may benefit from eliminating them.

One way to speed up the elimination of toxins through your lungs is to improve your breathing habits. It is worth spending a few minutes four or five times a day to do deep breathing exercises. Most people breathe shallowly and only fill up the top ¼ – ⅓ of their lungs. To learn how to breathe deeply using the full volume of your lungs, sit up straight, stand up or lie down, and place your hands on your lower rib cage at each side. As you breathe you should feel your hands are being pushed outwards as your rib cage swings out. Your chest is not meant to come up towards your chin. You should be breathing, moving your abdomen and not your chest. You can also place your hands on the portion of your lower rib cage nearest your spine and, if you can feel that portion swinging out, you know you have got it really right. By breathing deeply, ideally in through the nose and out through the mouth, you encourage the elimination of toxins through your breath. Deep breathing also promotes blood circulation in the organs of the abdomen, including the liver, as the diaphragm massages the area. An advanced option which has an even more potent effect on cleansing the liver, is to continue lowering the abdomen after you have exhaled. By pulling the muscles of the stomach in you get an even more powerful massage of the abdominal organs.

Part Three

TIME FOR ACTION

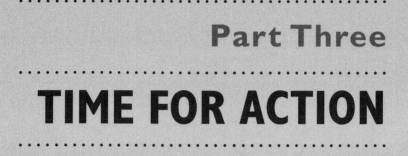

CHAPTER FIVE

Help Your Liver

The liver is really quite forgiving – despite the fact that we usually take it for granted. The liver deals with harmful compounds, sacrifices some of its fabric when proteins are needed elsewhere, and stores toxins when they have nowhere else to go. Despite the fact that we ask it to deal with alcohol, a high-fat and sugar diet, which play havoc with its chemistry, it is an organ that has an astounding ability to regenerate itself. If you give it what it needs, in terms of nutrients, reducing its workload and giving it a rest from time to time, it can repay you by carrying out vital, but silent, activities with maximum efficiency. Ensuring optimal nourishment can help to produce results in a reasonable period of time. The time depends on the individual's make up, and how much damage needs to be undone, but impressive results can usually begin to be felt in a few weeks.

Some suggested programmes to support your liver and speed up detoxification, are covered in **Three Plans**, page 72, but we will start with an overview of the key points for encouraging liver health.

You will have guessed by now that it is best to minimise your intake of, or preferably cut out altogether, stimulants such as alcohol, caffeine and sugar (see **Clean Up Your Act**, page 126). Healthy eating can give a natural 'high' which reduces your dependency on artificial boosts. If it is sweetness you crave, you will get a longer-lasting fix from fruit smoothies, or chunks of sweet tasting fruits such as watermelon, bananas, plums, peaches, grapes or kiwis. A drink of fresh fruit juice with sparkling water can be a refreshing alternative to wine with a meal, and

there are many delicious fruit and herbal teas which are caffeine
free.

Make a point of increasing your intake of all fruit and vegetables, especially those that are rich in antioxidants, as these
have a profound effect on liver functioning. Fruit and vegetables
with deep colours such as carrots, tomatoes, peppers, watercress, berries, beetroot and dark grapes have these beneficial
qualities (see Three Plans, page 72). It is also advantageous to eat
cruciferous vegetables, such as broccoli, cauliflower, Brussels
sprouts, cabbage, kohlrabi and kale, as these contain isothio-
cyanates and flavanoids which are potent P450 enzyme support-
ers. Feast on main meal salads, vegetarian meal options, delicious fruit salads and vegetable soups to increase your intake.
Eating this way need not take a lot of time. For instance, keep
lentil, and other soups, in the fridge or freezer and eat them with
a side salad of tomatoes and freshly cut basil or tarragon drizzled
with cold-pressed olive oil, or hummus served with cucumber,
carrot and celery sticks and broccoli florets. A meal such as this
is both filling and satisfying, can be made in ten minutes, and is
loaded with antioxidants and liver supporting compounds.

Eat healthy fats, as these can help to build healthy liver cells.
Sources include oily fish, such as tuna, salmon, mackerel, sar-
dines, anchovies and shark, as well as fresh unroasted, unsalted
nuts and seeds, and nut and seed butters. Use (cold pressed) olive
oil to cook with, and olive, flax or walnut oils for salads (again,
always use those that are cold pressed). Reduce your intake of
meat fat, butter, cream, cheese and full fat milk, and cut out margarines and heated vegetable oils such as corn and sunflower oil.

Reducing your dependency on processed foods is the only
way to avoid the majority of additives that find their way on to
the plate, including the very high amounts of sugar, salt and
hydrogenated fats, as well as cheap 'filler' ingredients. Take
delight in preparing more meals from fresh ingredients and

make a point of practising with one new recipe a week to build up your repertoire.

Drink plenty of filtered or mineral water – at least 2 litres a day (see **The Purest Drink of All?**, page 118). Jazz your water up by adding lemon juice, fresh fruit juices and herbs. Use fruit and herb teas (hot or chilled) or home-made cordials prepared with fructose (fruit sugar) instead of table sugar.

Avoid chemicals whenever possible, for example cigarette smoke and exhaust fumes, and eat organic food to reduce your exposure to pesticides. For a more detailed discussion on this, see **Clean Up Your Act**, page 126.

Avoid over-the-counter medications, and speak to your doctor about the necessity of taking prescribed medication, especially if you are on multiple medication. Discuss with him or her the possibility of obtaining non-toxic alternatives to the medication via, for instance, a herbalist or nutritionist, but do not stop prescribed medication without your doctor's permission. You may find that, as a by-product of your general detoxification programme, you are no longer dependent upon some types of medication, such as painkillers.

Some substances, which might normally be thought of as healthy, can have an adverse effect if your P450 enzyme balance is compromised (see **Love Your Liver**, page 23). While B-vitamins are generally helpful for speeding up detoxification, if an imbalance between Phases 1 and 2 exists, taking B-vitamins may make the situation worse rather than better because they rev up the Phase 1 stage, leaving the Phase 2 stage less able to cope. A substance called narangenin, found in grapefruit, can significantly inhibit the P450 enzymes. The same is not true of oranges and lemons, and the compound limonene found in these is helpful. If you are taking the nutrional trace mineral molybdenum, which is needed for optimal health, it competes with sulphate and may be best avoided if your P450 enzymes are not working properly.

Three Plans

Now that we have covered the basic theory behind the body's detoxification mechanisms, and explored some ways of accelerating the detox process, it is time for real action! This section contains three possible plans for you to follow, all of which can be adapted to suit your particular needs. The following is a brief summary of what they entail:

The Three-day Intensive Detox

This can be used as an occasional spring-clean, as a regular part of your health programme, say once monthly, or as an introduction to the longer-term detox programmes.

The Ten-day Fix

This is a more sustained approach to detoxification, which therefore produces more long-term results. It is an excellent introduction to the subject of healthy eating.

The Long-life Plan

It is important to recognise that it is long-term changes to eating habits which yield the best results. Once you have got used to some of the principles of eating to maximise your body's ability to deal with toxins, this approach is one you may like to use for life.

Read through the plans to help you to decide which approach most appeals to you, which is workable within the context of your life, and which is most likely to reap health benefits for you. Whichever one you choose, it is best to plan well ahead when embarking on a detox plan, for a variety of reasons. You may find that you need to juggle your dietary needs with those of your family, or that in order to avoid going off the rails in the middle of your detox, it is best for you not to visit a supermarket laden with temptations. Apart from buying in foods for your store cupboard, and shopping for fresh items, you can also decide in advance on your meal plans, using those given in this book as your starting point.

Supermarkets have finally caught on to the fact that there is a growing interest in healthy eating, and you can usually find a reasonable supply of organic fruit, vegetables, dairy produce, meats and other products at any large store. There are also many excellent independent suppliers of organic produce, and these are often much cheaper than the supermarkets, particularly if you live in the country. Many will have a box scheme available, which also eliminates the need for tedious shopping. Health food shops are the best source of alternative food substitutes, though do not assume that all the foods they stock are healthy. Many so-called healthy foods are just as laden with sugars and hydrogenated fats as the 'normal' varieties and you need to read the labels, just as you would in the supermarket, to familiarise yourself with the ingredients. It is also possible to order a wide range of organic and speciality foods via the internet, to be delivered within 48 hours. They tend to be more expensive, but save both on petrol and time and, in addition, prevent any impulse purchases you might make when you visit shops or supermarkets. The **Resources** section at the end of the book lists some suggestions for speciality foods (such as gluten-free foods) as a starting point.

You may also find it worthwhile to invest in a water filter, a juicer for hard fruits and vegetables (such as apples and carrots), and either a number of glass jars, or a sprouter, in which to sprout grains, seeds and nuts. If you really enjoy eating for a toxic-free life, you could also invest in a dehydrator to make a range of delicious dried biscuits and other snacks.

Of course, it is not necessary to go out and spend a fortune just because you are embarking on a detox. Indeed, the very idea of getting in special equipment may put you off. Many people, however, have an expensive food processor sitting unused at the back of the cupboard, and this is the perfect opportunity to dust it off and bring it back in to service!

The following is a brief list of possible aids for a 'natural-kitchen':

- **food processor** This is an essential piece of equipment for the healthy kitchen. With it you can chop and grate vegetables in seconds to make a range of delicious and appealing salads and soup ingredients.
- **blender** A blender is not vital if you have a food processor, but it is just a little bit easier to make fruit smoothies in it. To soft fruit, such as bananas, strawberries or peaches, add water or milk (soya, rice or oat milks are best) and then add nutrient boosters such as wheatgerm (though not if you are hypersensitive to wheat), a tiny bit of molasses, vitamin C powder, or lecithin and some flax oil.
- **mouli or grater** This is a useful bit of kit for making morning muesli. The perfect muesli, which is based on the original recipe for this popular dish and is called Bircher muesli, bears no relationship to the box of grains on the supermarket shelves. The ideal muesli involves soaking two or three tablespoons of oats overnight in fruit juice or water to break down some of the more indigestible carbo-

hydrates. After soaking the oats, add chopped dried fruit such as apricots, figs and raisins, and seeds such as pumpkin, sunflower and linseeds. Finally, when you are ready to eat it, grate an apple into the mixture, using your mouli or grater, then add a little yoghurt. The mixture ends up being more fruit than grains, which is probably a better balance for most people. It is moist and utterly delicious!

- **juicer** The most useful juicers are those which can deal with hard vegetables and fruits such as carrots and apples. They can be bought fairly inexpensively from most department stores, but the really professional non-centrifugal model is only available from a speciality supplier (listed in **Resources**, page 175). Juicing is both quick and easy, and the most difficult part is choosing which delicious juice you are going to make. If you get in the habit of washing your produce when you first buy it and before you store it in the fridge, you can make a juice with little preparation time. To avoid difficult cleaning of your juicer, plunge the removable parts of the machine into a sink of clean water immediately after making your juice and you will find that cleaning it takes no time at all.

- **sprouting jars** Sprouts can be made from all sorts of beans, pulses, lentils, nuts and seeds. The best ones to experiment with are: sunflower seeds, pumpkin seeds, almonds, aduki beans, mung beans, alfalfa, chickpeas, lentils, whole oats or buckwheat. You do not need to buy sprouting jars to do this as you can use any fairly large clear glass container, covering the top with a square of muslin or even kitchen paper, secured with an elastic band. However, if you find that you enjoy eating sprouts, which are some of the most potent detoxifiers, a set of sprouting jars is a neat and attractive addition to your kitchen and one that makes the whole process just that little more appealing.

First discard any broken or damaged beans, seeds, nuts or grains, then soak them in filtered water for 12–24 hours and then drain. Leave the covered jar in a warm, dark place for two to five days, depending on what you are sprouting, until you get the length of sprout you require. During this time make sure that you rinse and drain the sprouts twice a day. When they are long enough, place the jar on a windowsill for the sprouts to catch the light and turn green. Continue to rinse and drain them twice daily. When they turn green they are ready to eat, at which point they can be kept in the fridge for a few days.

● **dehydrator** This is the least necessary addition to your kitchen, but it is simplicity itself to use (and considerably easier than cooking). A dehydrator is like a small oven, but it does not allow food to heat up above 110 degrees Fahrenheit. Instead, it gently dehydrates it over a 12–24 hour period, allowing you to create a range of delicious dried snacks. The advantage of these foods is that they are easy to prepare, and they retain the nutritional advantages of raw foods. To this end they can be a real boon in a detoxification programme. Dried biscuits and snacks can be made from ground sunflower seeds, sprouted chickpeas and sprouted grains such as oats and buckwheat. They can be made savoury with the addition of tomato and garlic or curry and coriander, or sweet with the addition of honey, dates or apricots. Home-made dried fruits, which are preservative free, are easy to make, muesli bars are delicious, and dried vegetables, such as mushrooms and dried tomatoes, make tasty additions to soups.

THE THREE-DAY INTENSIVE DETOX

The Three-day Intensive Detox is really a modified fast. Most fasts consist of avoiding all food, while drinking copious amounts of water, or drinking fruit or vegetable juices (juice fast) or eating as much of a single fruit as is desired (mono-fruit fast). Such fasts must not be followed for more than a day or two without professional supervision; more information about them is given in **Fasting**, page 149. It is, however, quite appropriate for most people to follow a modified fast along the lines of that described below. The advantage is that you need not go hungry and you can eat as much as you like of the selected foods. Most people find they are perfectly capable of carrying on with their normal routine during the Three-day Intensive Detox, though it is probably best to do it over a long weekend, when you can rest a little more than normal, and are not subject to the stresses of a normal working day.

The Three-day Intensive Detox can be used:

● **as a spring clean** – a 'pick-me-up' once or twice a year
● **as a regular body workout** – a monthly clear out
● **for ultimate reconditioning** – as a boost before The Ten-day Fix followed by The Long-life Plan.

The aim of the regime is to give your body a chance to recuperate – a sort of weekend holiday for the digestive system and the liver. Giving your liver a break from having to do too much digestive work processing difficult substances such as lots of proteins or alcohol enables it to concentrate on dealing with previously accumulated debris, and allows it an opportunity to regenerate itself. Of course, true regeneration can only take place over a longer period, by following the Long-life Plan, but this is a pretty good place for most people to start.

Who should not do the Three-day Intensive Detox?

Do not do this short, sharp Three-day Detox, or indeed any other detox, if you are pregnant or breast feeding. The reason for this is that, even though this plan involves eating healthy foods, you will release stored toxins into your system which could have a detrimental effect on the baby. If you are ill, under medical supervision, are very underweight, are diabetic, or have an eating disorder, you are best advised to get medical advice about following a detox plan. Most people will benefit from a detox, but if your system is already weakened, you should not go it alone with such a plan. Many people will find that they experience unpleasant symptoms, sometimes quite severe, from detoxification. This does not mean that they should not go ahead with a detox, but that they may need to adopt a slower approach by using the Ten-day Fix or the Long-life Plan instead. The symptoms that indicate you are off-loading toxins include headaches, furred up tongue, spots, a change in body odour, cloudy urine and a change in bowel habits. None of these symtons should persist, however. You may also feel more tired than usual, and it is best to give in to the need to nap or sleep to conserve your body's energy. It is also a good idea to keep warm and to do a little gentle exercise, such as walking, but to not overtax yourself. Eating lots of vegetables, if you are unused to it, may lead to some digestive problems, in which case you may also need to take the slower approach to detoxing. It is always helpful to incorporate other means of speeding up elimination of toxins from the body while following a detox programme, so give yourself a daily dry skin brush (see page 54), have a massage or visit an acupuncturist or reflexologist who can use techniques to help the process along, though discuss what you are planning to do with them before making your appointment.

The eating plan

The eating plan below is designed to give you some ideas about how to follow a Three-day Intensive Detox. Once you become used to following such a plan, you do not need to stick to it slavishly, but can make up your own recipes, as long as you respect the basic guidelines listed below detailing what you can, and cannot, have. You will see that many fruit-based snacks have been included, and this is to keep you from feeling hungry. Again, you do not have to follow this slavishly. You can eat snacks at any time – you may even find that you need to eat a piece of fruit, or drink a fresh fruit or vegetable juice, or cup of home-made vegetable soup, every hour. If you find that you must work during your detox, this can easily be accommodated by taking fruit, juices or a flask of soup into work to snack on regularly, and by ensuring that your main meal consists of a huge salad. Make sure that you stay well hydrated while following this plan, and drink a large glass of water every hour, or even every half hour. You can enhance the cleansing effect of the programme if you start your day by drinking the juice of half a lemon diluted with warm filtered water. Make a tea twice a day using a teaspoonful of chopped dandelion root, simmered gently in a mugful of filtered water for 15 minutes. Alternatively, use a liquid artichoke or dandelion based detox formula.

When you have finished your Three-day Intensive Detox, ease back into eating 'normally'. Do not make your first meal a huge fry-up with all the trimmings! Your stomach will only rebel. Instead go for something such as stir-fried vegetables with shredded chicken or tofu, a vegetable filled wholemeal pitta pocket, or a thick lentil or bean soup.

What you can have
All fruits, including exotic fruit and fresh fruit cocktails.

Vegetables, including steamed, stir-fried or baked vegetables, sprouted grains, nuts and seeds and vegetable juices, vegetable broths, herbal teas, brown rice (and rice milk), quinoa, millet, corn, buckwheat, fresh raw nuts and seeds. The majority of foods are best eaten raw or lightly steamed to get the most enzymes out of them and to put the least pressure on the liver. In addition to the fats found in fresh nuts and seeds, avocados, fresh coconut and tahini, allow yourself half a tablespoon of olive oil and half a tablespoon of flax oil daily. Use loads of flavourings such as garlic and fresh herbs.

What you must not have
No alcohol, coffee, tea, sugar, salt, processed foods, dairy produce, wheat or meat whatsoever.

Supplements
Do not take supplements during a short, sharp detox such as this, as they need to be processed by the liver and it is best to let it rest as much as possible. Keep supplements for the longer, more gentle, detoxes.

Three-day Intensive Detox shopping list

In order to make the most of your detox weekend, it is best to prepare ahead. To help you to do this, I have compiled a complete shopping list of all the ingredients you will need. I have not repeated this for the other programmes, since you can base your planning for them on this list, adding foods you enjoy that fit in with the particular plan you are following. Ingredients such as seaweed or tamari, which may be unfamiliar to some of you, can easily be obtained from good quality health food shops (or see **Resources**, page 171).

store cupboard ingredients

apricots, dried (preferably unsulphured)
brown rice
cayenne pepper
coconut
cumin
dulse flakes (seaweed)
garlic

Hijiki seaweed (optional)
millet flakes
paprika
quinoa
tamari
turmeric
vanilla extract

fridge

almonds, flaked and ground
flax oil (cold-pressed, organic)
olive oil (cold-pressed, organic)
olives, black

pecans
pine nuts
rice milk
sesame seeds
tahini

freezer ingredients

frozen berries (ideally mixed)

fruit

1 apple, cooking
1 apple, dessert
3 apricots
1 avocado
3 bananas, small
1 grapefruit
1 grapes, red, small bunch
1 kiwi

3 lemons
1 lime
1 mango
1 orange
1 papaya
1 pear
1 tangerine
1 watermelon, small

vegetables

1 packet alfalfa sprouts	1 pepper, red
1 beetroot	1 pepper, yellow
1 broccoli floret	2 potatoes, large
6 carrots	½ pumpkin
1 celery head	1 bunch radishes
½ cucumber	1 red onion
1 cob of corn (frozen if	1 bunch spring onions
necessary)	2 sweet potatoes
1 fennel	8 tomatoes, medium large

garden or pots on windowsill

basil	parsley
mint	rosemary

AND HERE IS THE PLAN – ENJOY IT!

SNACK: Watermelon Juice

Liquidise the flesh of a watermelon, making sure you include the seeds. If you are using a juicer you can include some of the (scrubbed) rind as well.

Day Three

BREAKFAST: Vanilla Smoothie

1 tbsp tahini
2 small bananas
vanilla extract
½ cup water (more if you like a thinner consistency)

Millet Porridge

Made with water or rice milk and chopped dried fruit.

SNACK: Fresh fruit

Large slice of watermelon

LUNCH: Technicolour Jacket Potato

Arrange the following rainbow salad around a jacket potato:

red: grated beetroot
white: grated radish
orange: grated carrot
green: handful of chopped parsley
yellow: yellow pepper
black: olives

and sprinkle with paprika, lemon juice and ½ tbsp flax oil.

SNACK: Square Fruit

Cubed mango, lime juice and chopped pecans

EVENING: Tomato and Basil Soup

Liquidise or juice six large skinned tomatoes. Add the juice of
¼ of a lemon, a splash of tamari and a pinch of dulse flakes
(seaweed). Finally, stir in 1 tbsp of chopped fresh basil.
Serve either hot or cold.

Corn on the Cob

with olive oil and garlic and freshly ground black pepper

SNACK: Almond Baked Apple

Fill a large, cored cooking apple with almond apricot filling:
3 finely chopped dried apricots (or other dried fruit)
mixed to a paste with 2 tsp ground almonds and 1–2 tsp
almond butter and a splash of warm water. Bake in a hot
oven for 20 minutes and sprinkle with flaked almonds and
mixed spice for the last 5 minutes of baking.

THE TEN-DAY FIX

Whereas the Three-day Intensive Detox is a useful short-term or
kick-start detox, the Ten-day Fix is a way of easing yourself into
a lifetime of healthy eating. It is also the ideal way to clean out
your system before going on holiday or preparing yourself for a
special event, such as a family wedding or Christmas, when you
will need more reserves than usual. If you found the Three-day
Intensive Detox difficult because your adverse reactions were
too intense (from detoxifying too quickly) this slower approach
will probably suit you better.

The Ten-day Fix includes lots of vital, organic, healthy eating, and avoids the foods and drinks that are most likely to overtax the body's detoxification systems, such as excess fats, gluten
grains and dairy products. It focuses on fruit and vegetables,

gluten-free grains, seafood and lean meats, tofu, beans and pulses, plus healthy sources of fats such as nuts, seeds, avocados and olive oil. It is often the case on a healthy eating programme that you are required to 'breakfast like a king' by eating something carbohydrate-based. However, if you are aiming to detoxify, you may want to take a different approach, and instead extend the 'fast' of the night into the morning by eating a fruit-based breakfast that will not overtax your digestive system (this is not the same as skipping breakfast, which is not a good idea). If you feel hungry on such a regime, you can snack on as many fruits as you like throughout the morning until you reach lunchtime. Alternatively, if you are one of those people who definitely feel better after having a 'proper' breakfast of some grains, make sure that your selections are gluten-free grains, such as millet porridge, corn or quinoa flakes or breakfast rice (see page 98). To make a delicious topping for any breakfast cereal, blend a banana with some silken tofu and use this and fruit juice to moisten the cereal. Snacks have not been included in this programme, but eating fresh fruit, nuts, seeds and a small amount of dried fruit is ideal. Make sure that you continue to drink at least 2 litres of filtered water daily to keep flushing out the impurities which will be eliminated by following this programme.

Day One

BREAKFAST: Berry Whizz

Mixed berries (i.e. strawberries, blackberries, blueberries)
    whizzed in a liquidiser, with silken tofu.

LUNCH: Tofu and Mushroom Medley

Cook mushrooms, garlic and chives in a little olive oil. Add
tofu and tamari and serve with a green salad.

EVENING: Steamed Vegetable Platter

Steam new potatoes (small), whole carrots, beetroot cut in
quarters, broccoli florets, cauliflower florets and a quartered courgette. Garnish with fresh herbs and cherry
tomatoes. Serve with mackerel or salmon paté.

Day Two

BREAKFAST: Apple and Seed Crunch

Cooked puréed apple with cinnamon and 1–2 tbsp mixed
seeds (sunflower, pumpkin, sesame).

LUNCH: Grated Roots and Veggieburgers

Veggieburger: grated carrot (plus some extra for the salad),
diced onion, a large amount of chopped parsley and
thyme, millet flakes and roasted sesame seeds. Use enough
beaten egg to bind the ingredients together and season.
Shape into burgers, brush with olive oil and cook in a
medium oven for 40 minutes. Serve with grated carrot (or
sweet potato), grated beetroot and sweet corn.

EVENING: Paprika Chicken with Sage Butter (Lima) Beans

Chicken: sauté 5-cm chicken pieces with spring onions and
green pepper in a little olive oil, add chopped tomatoes
and paprika.
Butter beans with sage and garlic: sauté cooked beans in oil,
lemon juice, lemon zest and roughly chopped sage leaves.

Day Three

BREAKFAST: Prune and Apricot Compote

Stew dried prunes and apricots in a little water, then add soya
   yoghurt and chopped fresh nuts to serve.

LUNCH: Thick Spicy Leek and Potato Soup

Soften chopped leeks in oil, then add diced potato and just
   enough water to cover, and season with garlic, pepper,
   turmeric and cumin. When the potatoes are soft, blend
   until smooth. Serve with a sprinkling of grilled crispy
   bacon (no fat).

EVENING: Sprouted Bean Stir-fry with Brown Rice

Stir-fry onion, garlic, sprouts (i.e. sprouted lentils, mung beansprouts and/or alfalfa), mangetout, fennel, red pepper, red
   cabbage and water chestnuts. Add shredded cooked chicken
   if you wish. Season with tamari. Sprinkle liberally with
   sesame seeds and parsley and serve on a bed of brown rice.

Day Four

BREAKFAST: Mango Whizz

Mango flesh whizzed in a liquidiser, with silken tofu.

LUNCH: Herb Omelette with Fennel Salad

Fennel salad: chopped fennel, radish slices, cucumber and basil
   tossed in shredded leaves. Serve with a lemon dressing.

EVENING: Steamed Halibut with Capers and Tomato

Place the halibut in an ovenproof dish, cover with sliced
   tomatoes, garlic and capers. Sprinkle with cayenne pepper

and paprika. Cover and bake in a pre-heated medium oven for 15-20 minutes. Serve with steamed chard or spinach.

Day Five

BREAKFAST: Crunchy Spiced Banana
Mash or chop a banana with a sprinkling of ginger, then add mixed seeds and a handful of blueberries or other berries.

LUNCH: Prawn, Egg and Globe Artichoke Salad
Boil the artichoke for 30 minutes. Remove the outer leaves and coarse centre, then cut into wedges. (Alternatively, use canned artichoke hearts.) Soft boil an organic free-range egg, then cut that into wedges too, and place, with the artichoke, on a bed of shredded lettuce, chopped chives and shredded mint leaves, then add some black olives and cooked prawns. Serve with a sharp mint dressing made by whisking together olive oil, red wine vinegar, mustard, garlic and mint.

EVENING: Rainbow Rice
Sauté chopped red pepper, carrot, pumpkin, red cabbage and spring onions in olive oil. Add tamari sauce and 1 cup of cooked brown rice per person. Add enough water just to cover the bottom of the pan and leave to cook for 5 minutes. Add cayenne pepper and tofu as desired, plus a liberal amount of chopped parsley.

Day Six

BREAKFAST: Almond Apple
A baked apple stuffed with apricots and a teaspoon of almond butter.

LUNCH: Northern Beet Salad

Chop beetroot immediately after cooking. Leave in a marinade
of garlic and vinegar for 30 mins. Add finely chopped
spring onion, cucumber and fresh dill, and mix with a
small amount of natural live yoghurt. Finally add chopped
hard-boiled egg. Serve on green leaves drizzled with lemon
juice.

EVENING: Smoked Chicken and Tomato Salad

Roughly shred the chicken and toss into a salad made from
fresh leaves and herbs (rocket, baby cos, coriander, flat
leaf parsley, basil). Serve on a bed of sliced beef tomatoes
drizzled with a flax oil and balsamic dressing and sprinkle
with pine nuts.

Day Seven

BREAKFAST: Mulled Pears and Orange

Cut each pear into six wedges and divide the orange into segments. Place in a pan with a little water and some mixed
spice and gently warm. Add some whole almonds and
serve warm.

LUNCH: Baltic Soup

Soften chopped onion, diced carrot and turnip and shredded
cabbage in oil, then leave to steam for 15 minutes. Add
equal amounts of chickpeas, kidney beans and corn, then
cover with water, season with tamari and paprika, and
simmer for 10 minutes. Add a generous amount of
chopped parsley and serve.

EVENING: Barbecued Monkfish

Thread alternate chunks of monkfish and pineapple on to a

skewer and either barbecue or grill until browned. Serve with roasted vegetables and a green side salad.

Day Eight

BREAKFAST: Cashana

Blend 1 banana with ½–1 cup cashew nuts, plus a little water to mix, if necessary. Once blended, add a handful of whole frozen berries.

LUNCH: Spicy Nut Coleslaw and Baked Potato

Shred cabbage, carrot, apple and onion and toss in spicy dressing made from silken tofu, vinegar, oil, garlic, mustard and curry herbs. Add chopped walnuts and serve with a leaf salad and baked potato.

EVENING: Chicken and Red Pepper Casserole with Vegetables

Vegetables: broccoli, carrots, red onion, corn and arame seaweed (cooked for about 10 minutes). Serve with the chicken and red pepper casserole (skinned chicken portions, on the bone, slow-simmered for 1–1½ hours with onions, garlic, tomatoes, red pepper, mushrooms in salt free stock with some white wine – the alcohol will cook-off).

Day Nine

BREAKFAST: Fruit Kebabs

Thread alternate chunks of passion fruit, fresh pineapple and strawberries on to a skewer, then grill lightly on all sides. Eat with toasted almonds.

LUNCH: Tuna with Beany Watercress and Mushroom Salad

Make a salad from watercress, mung beansprouts (or other
sprouts), sliced button mushrooms, chopped parsley and
spring onions, add the tuna and drizzle with a spicy dressing made from lemon juice, flax oil, garlic and cayenne
pepper.

EVENING: Vegetarian Chilli

Soften some onion and garlic in oil. Add cooked brown lentils,
cooked kidney beans, chopped green pepper and celery,
tinned tomatoes, tomato purée, lemon juice, chilli powder,
cumin and basil. Serve with soya yoghurt and a green
salad.

Day Ten

BREAKFAST: Peach Whizz

Ripe peach flesh whizzed in a liquidiser with silken tofu.

LUNCH: Broccoli, Arame and Pecan Salad

Add soaked arame seaweed to steamed broccoli florets and
carrots cut into matchsticks. Add fanned avocado, then
sprinkle with toasted pecans and a tamari dressing and
serve.

**EVENING: Grilled Pesto Cod Served with Green and
Orange Vegetables**

Make a pesto using either pine or cashew nuts and basil,
substituting tofu for the cheese. Spread pesto liberally on
both sides of the fish fillet, then grill. Serve with runner
beans and mashed sweet potato.

. . . .

THE LONG-LIFE PLAN

One of the aims of both the Three-day Intensive Detox and the Ten-day Fix is to enable you to dip your toe in the water of dietary change and to introduce you to a life of reduced toxin exposure. When starting any new programme it takes time to learn the 'tricks of the trade', and the two earlier, shorter plans can help to do this. By now, hopefully, you will be committed to making longer-term changes to your lifestyle. It is always best to start slowly and to build up to altering the way you do things. If you jump in too enthusiastically there is always the danger that you will find the changes too difficult. Better to allow your healthy diet to evolve gradually and to make changes that become a normal and unstressful part of your daily life.

The Long-life Plan is all about learning to eat a healthy diet for the long-term. Outlined below are a number of suggestions for meals and snacks, but you will no doubt learn to adapt recipes to your own taste. Just remember to keep to the following important guidelines:

- Base your meals on fruit, vegetables, beans, pulses, nuts and seeds, at the same time keeping your intake of gluten grains and dairy produce to a minimum. Use goat's and sheep's milk products in preference to cow's milk ones.
- Make sure that your fats come from healthy sources, including cold pressed oils such as olive, flax, walnut and sunflower oil, and from fresh nuts and seeds, avocados, coconut and oily fish.
- Drink 2 litres (8–10 large glasses) of filtered water daily.
- Keep your exposure to toxins from food additives, chemicals, coffee and alcohol to a minimum.
- Choose a good fibre powder or supplement, such as psyllium husks, pectin or linseeds (whole seeds ground up), to keep your digestive tract in good working order and to

keep toxins moving out of your body.

● Incorporate regular 'body work' into your routine –
exercise, massage, saunas, skin brushing (see page 54).

● Occasionally do a modified fast (using the Three-day
Intensive Detox).

● If you are inclined to take supplements to speed up
detoxification, make sure that your supplement plan
includes the following:
  – the antioxidant vitamins: vitamin A 15,000 ius, vitamin
  E 300 mg, vitamin C 2 g (1 g twice daily)
  – a high strength mineral formula that includes the
  minerals most important for detoxification: zinc 20 mg,
  selenium 100–200 mcg, calcium 500 mg, magnesium
  350–500 mg, iron 10 mg, manganese 5–10 mg
  – one of the liver support herbs, such as milk thistle or
  dandelion

optional
  – antioxidant enzyme support nutrients such as N-acetyle
  cysteine 200 mg or one of the special liver support
  formulas that include the sulphur amino acids
  – garlic, seaweed/kelp or chlorella/spirulina supplements
  (see **Heavy Metals**, page 140).

Short cuts

To add to your new repertoire, here are a few short cuts and
strategies to help make your life easier and to ensure that you
are not caught short when in a hurry – because that is the time
when you are most likely to go for what is quick and easy. If
what you have available is health promoting, you win on all
fronts.

● Aim to keep assorted greens, red peppers, fresh herbs, olives and root vegetables handy in your fridge. This way you can always throw together a quick meal. Buy the freshest organic produce you can find and shop twice a week. If you wash most of the produce before you put it in the fridge, you can prepare a meal in a matter of minutes instead of having to scrub vegetables for ages.

● If you do not already have one, invest in a food processor. With it you can do any of the following in no time at all:
– shred cabbage, carrots and onions to make a large coleslaw (use yoghurt and vinaigrette for the dressing).
– whip up a thick and nourishing soup
– make a bean paté, guacamole or a tapenada (to make the latter, use one, two or all of the following: pitted black olives, anchovies, sun-dried tomatoes. Blend with a little olive oil, basil leaves and some Parmesan; it will last for up to a week in the fridge)
– whizz up a luxurious fresh fruit pudding using tofu.

● If you keep any dressing on the side, salads will stay fresh in the fridge for an instant solution to your next meal.

● Keep a couple of types of sprouts in your fridge at any one time to add to salads or sandwiches, sprinkle on soups or to have as snacks. Ideally, make them yourself using sprouting jars (see **Three Plans**, page 75), but if this isn't possible, mung beansprouts and alfalfa sprouts are usually readily available in the chill cabinet of good health food shops.

● Keep a number of foods in the freezer so that you never run out, and they remain at peak freshness. Some which you might not have thought of keeping there include:
– pre-cooked beans, kept in portion sizes, to add to soups, salads, to use as a side dish (dressed with oil and lemon) or to make a dip

– pre-cooked brown rice, in portion sizes, to use with main courses, to add to salads, or to make breakfast rice (defrost the night before and add warm soya milk, chopped nuts, seeds, dried fruit, grated apple, mashed bananas or coconut cream or flakes)

– bananas freeze well – but peel and store in a container first – then whizz up with berries and goat's milk (or other milk) while frozen for an instant frozen pudding or defrost them and add to cereals, yoghurt or other dishes

– keep containers of frozen berries to add to breakfast dishes or puddings

– keep pre-chopped herbs loosely frozen to add to dishes to give instant jazz to your cooking

– keep shelled nuts, seeds, coconut and dried fruit in the freezer to keep them fresh

– freshly made, thick vegetable and bean soups kept in portion sizes will help to keep you on track.

● Make dishes that will keep well for several days in the fridge, to dip into at those snacky moments. Sauerkraut keeps for ages, as do pickles, and bean dips and olives will stay fresh for several days. Salad dressings also last for quite a while, so you can keep a few choices (tahini, herb, balsamic, honey and lemon), depending on your mood and what you want to dip into them

● Plain, live yoghurt kept in the fridge is great to add at the last minute to soups and other dishes to give them a creamy texture, also to make a low-fat coleslaw dressing, to jazz up baked potatoes, to add to salad dressings or use as a dessert with chopped nuts and dried or fresh fruit.

7 Breakfast Ideas

Soya Yoghurt and Fruit
Live soya yoghurt, with sliced pear and pumpkin seeds.

Citrus Medley
Grapefruit and orange segments.

Boiled Eggs

Gluten-free Muesli with Sheep's Yoghurt
Muesli: a combination of soya flakes, rice flakes, buckwheat
groats with unsulphured dried apricots and prunes, and
almonds, coconut shavings and pumpkin seeds.

Apricot Whizz
Whizz together tofu and fresh ripe apricot halves in a
liquidiser — adjusting the proportion of fruit to tofu to
taste — and add mint leaves and sharon fruit (optional).

Breakfast Rice with Tahini
Stir cooked brown rice and a little water over a medium heat.
As it thickens, add a little tahini to taste, plus some
cinnamon. Serve with toasted sesame seeds, hazelnuts and
soaked dried prunes.

Banana
Baked banana with cinnamon and yoghurt.

Cornflakes or Rice Puffs
With either soya milk or fruit.

7 Snack Ideas

Crispy Chinese Seeds
Toast sunflower seeds that have been tossed in tamari sauce and store in a glass jar.

Bean Spread on Rice Cakes
Bean Spread: process or mash together cooked beans and chopped onion with a little olive oil, lemon juice and garlic, then flavour with fresh herbs and spices of your choice.

Frozen Banana
Peel a banana, cut in half, then roll each half, until covered, in crushed nuts and toasted sesame seeds. Put in a plastic container and place in the freezer. Ready to eat from frozen when peckish!

Fruit (Pick of the Bunch)
Portable: whole fruit, i.e. apples, pears, tangerines, apricots, plums, grapes, star fruit, bananas, etc.
At home: oranges cut into quarters, melon slices, pineapple rings, kiwi, mango, papaya, avocado, etc.

Home-made Fruit and Nut Mix
Mix almonds, sunflower seeds, pumpkin seeds, hazelnuts, pine nuts and pecans in a glass jar, then add unsweetened coconut shavings, unsulphured dried apricots and raisins and dried dates (no added glucose). Grab a palmful when you need a nibble.

Seaweed and Sesame Rice Crackers with Hummus Dip

Julienne Vegetables and Mackerel Pâté Dip
Mackerel pâté: blend mackerel, tofu, lemon juice and coarsely
    ground black pepper in a liquidiser until smooth.

Light Meal Ideas

Alfalfa and Runner Bean Salad with Tuna
Include black olives, plum tomatoes and mixed leaves in the
    salad. Serve with a flax oil and cider vinegar dressing.

Cabbage Borscht
Cook beetroot with potatoes for 20 minutes. Add cabbage,
    onion, celery, dill weed, vinegar, black pepper and tomato
    purée, and cook for a further 30 minutes. When ready,
    purée in a blender and serve drizzled with yoghurt.

Corn Pasta and Chickpea Salad
Toss cooked corn pasta, chickpeas, chopped red onion and
    chopped tomato in a vinaigrette dressing. Serve on a bed of
    baby spinach leaves, dandelion leaves and sliced fresh
    radishes.

Stuffed Red Peppers
Soften garlic, onion, celery and green pepper in oil. Add
    oregano, tamari, paprika, basil and pepper. Mix with
    cooked millet, rice or buckwheat and add tahini. Stuff red
    peppers with the filling and bake for 20–30 minutes.

Gazpacho Salad and Baked Potato
Finely chop parsley, red pepper, courgette, celery, cucumber
    and red onion. Add sweetcorn kernels. Fill the baked
    potato and dress with a ginger and lime dressing.

Hot Turkey Breast on a bed of Watercress and Tomato Salad

Roast turkey breast with thyme and lemon. When cooked, cut
into 4–5 diagonal pieces and place on a bed of watercress,
tomato and green olives. Serve with a peppered orange
and flax oil dressing

Rice-Baked-Beans

Heat equal weights of cooked black-eyed beans (or soya beans)
and cooked brown rice with garlic, diced onion and a can
of tomatoes (in concentrated tomato juice). Add mustard
and a splash of Worcestershire Sauce. Serve with mashed
swede and spring greens.

Crispy Bacon and Avocado Salad

Cut off all the fat from bacon rashers and grill. Add this to a
large green salad with chopped avocado and halved cherry
tomatoes.

Home-made Salmon Fish Cakes with Salad

Fish cakes: mix mashed potato, fresh or tinned salmon,
chopped capers and parsley, dulse flakes and coarsely
ground pepper. Shape, brush with olive oil, and put under
the grill until warmed through and brown. Serve with
tossed leaves and a cucumber and mint salad.

Lucky Dip – Day Out Clean-finger Lunch

Carrot sticks, celery sticks, cucumber sticks, radishes, grapes,
green olives, feta cheese and chicken cubes.

Mexican Salad Bowl

Toss shredded green lettuce, black-eyed beans, red onions,
cucumber, radishes and plum tomatoes in a Mexican

dressing (skinned and finely chopped tomatoes, finely chopped spring onions, garlic, olive oil, tamari and a touch of chilli).

Mackerel Asparagus Salad

Toss lightly cooked asparagus into a salad consisting of rocket, chicory, spring onions and herb leaves. Serve with peppered mackerel and basil vinaigrette.

Mushrooms on Toast

Soften onions in olive oil, add quartered mushrooms, then pour over a white sauce made from soya milk and the juice from the mushrooms and onions. Serve on rye toast with a liberal sprinkling of chopped parsley.

Lentil Pâté with Crackers

Lentil pâté: weigh equal amounts of cooked brown lentils and raw mushrooms. Cook the sliced mushrooms with garlic and finely chopped onion, then add the cooked lentils and some tamari and parsley. Blend in food processor, adding a little water if necessary. Season. Side salad: multi-coloured salad vegetables.

Main Meal Ideas

Polenta with Lentil and Tomato Sauce

Add cooked brown lentils to a home-made garlic bolognese (lots of fresh basil). Serve on polenta grain (cooked with 3 times the volume of water to maize meal). Serve with a green salad.

Baked Dill Salmon with Green Bean and Carrot Hash Browns

Carrot hash browns: finely grate carrot, onion and potato. Mix
together and flatten into a shallow cake tin, brush with
olive oil and cook in a hot oven until brown.

Sweet and Sour Chinese Cabbage

Lightly stir-fry roughly chopped cabbage, onion and (fresh)
pineapple cubes. Then pour over the sauce. Serve with
roasted buckwheat groats.

The sauce: mix together cornflour, olive oil, red hot pepper,
grated ginger, tamari and vinegar, then, just before serving,
add some walnut halves.

Traditional Roast Chicken

Before roasting the chicken, insert pieces of garlic into 6 x 1 cm
slits in thighs and breast, and add sprigs of rosemary and
thyme.

When cooked, serve with wakame carrots (steamed carrots
mixed with cooked wakame seaweed) and Brussels
sprouts.

Steamed Halibut in a Herb Marinade

Marinade: majoram, thyme, olive oil, lemon, balsamic vinegar.
Serve with lightly steamed yellow and green vegetables.

Winter Stir-fry Tofu with Quinoa

Vegetables: broccoli, cauliflower, parsnip and roughly sliced
red pepper.

Herbs: garlic, ginger, coriander.

Tofu: firm tofu cut into cubes.

Serve topped with toasted sesame seeds.

Fresh Tuna Niçoise

Make a salad of endive and chicory, then place green beans,
spring onions, black olives, cherry tomatoes, sliced boiled
egg, anchovies and new potatoes on top. Finally, add
chunks of lightly cooked fresh tuna. Serve with lots of
black pepper and a flax oil vinaigrette.

Pasta with Pesto

Mix together cooked buckwheat pasta, pesto, black olives,
finely chopped red pepper and small chunks of goat's
cheese. Sprinkle with pine nuts.

Curried Chickpeas and Brown Rice

Lightly fry onions and garlic. Stir in a small amount of cornflour or buckwheat flakes to thicken. Immediately add
chopped tomatoes, cooked chickpeas, spices and raisins.
Finally, add apple chunks and fresh coriander leaves. Serve
with brown rice.

Turkey with Warmed Pickled Cabbage and Peas

Mix chunks of turkey roasted with rosemary and orange with
cabbage and minted peas, and serve with an olive oil and
vinegar dressing and walnuts.

Nut Loaf

Blend or finely mince 500 g lightly toasted seeds and nuts
(sunflower seeds, hazelnuts and cashew nuts). Stir in a
chopped hard-boiled egg, lightly fried onion and finely
sliced celery. Bake in a shallow cake tin in a pre-heated
medium oven for 20–30 minutes. You can also add 250 g
cooked quinoa or barley to the mixture to vary the texture. Serve with steamed carrots and steamed kale with
caraway seeds.

Nori Parcels of White Fish

Poach fish wrapped in softened sheets of Nori seaweed. Serve
with sweet potato, steamed broccoli and a warmed tomato
and dill salad with a tamari dressing. Sprinkle with toasted
sesame seeds.

Prawns Tossed in a Green Sea

Stir-fry prawns and garlic, mangetout, spring onion, chinese
leaves and chopped mushrooms. Serve with brown rice or
quinoa.

Lime Salmon Fillets with Runner Beans, Roasted Fennel and New Potatoes

Lime salmon fillets: marinade the fillets in lime juice, finely
grated zest of lime and dill for 6 hours. Remove from the
marinade, brush with olive oil and grill until brown. To
serve, pour heated lime and dill juice over the fish and
sprinkle with coarsely ground black pepper.

CHAPTER SEVEN

Nature's Helping Hand

Herbs have been used for thousands of years to reduce 'biliousness' and 'liverishness'. Those which are bitter tasting often have the most potent effect. Many herbs contain compounds that directly influence liver and gall bladder function, and are generally divided into 'hepatics' and 'cholagogues'. Hepatic simply means liver, whereas cholagogues stimulate the flow of bile from the liver.

Common herbs and foods that significantly support liver function, and which can be liberally added to salads, soups and other dishes, include garlic, dandelion, chicory, lemon balm, artichoke, sage, rosemary, turmeric and butternut. Liver-supporting teas can also be made from a number of herbs such as thyme, rosemary, chamomile, meadowsweet and vervaine. All of the brassica family, including broccoli, Brussels sprouts, cabbage, cauliflower and kale, help to activate the P450 enzyme system responsible for liver detoxification.

Detox superfoods

A number of foods contain compounds that have been shown to improve liver and gall bladder action, cleanse blood, support the kidneys, and so support detoxification. This is not a finite list (others are covered throughout this chapter) but they are some of the most straightforward to ease into your eating plan.

artichokes globe artichakes contain cynarin, which stimulates the liver and gall bladder and promotes the digestion of fats

asparagus contains aspartic acid, which stimulates the kidneys and is mildly diuretic in action; also high in potassium, which rids the body of fluid retention

broccoli the compounds in this vegetable, and in the rest of the brassica family (cabbage, cauliflower, Brussels sprouts, kale, kholrabi), support the liver's detoxification enzymes

chicory the bitter tasting component, intybin, has a restorative effect on the liver and gall bladder, and stimulates digestion and metabolism

fennel the strong tasting oils in this bulb stimulate the liver and the kidneys and help digestion

garlic this herb, along with other members of the onion family, has potent blood cleansing properties

horseradish stimulates the gall bladder and kidneys, and has a mildly diuretic action

kohlrabi stimulates the flow of bile and supports the kidneys

leeks mustard oils stimulate the liver, gall bladder and kidneys, and potassium helps to deal with fluid retention; also rich in mucilage compounds, which cleanse the digestive tract

lovage cleanses and purifies the blood, stimulates the flow of bile and supports the kidneys

nettles excellent for de-acidifying body tissues as they arc highly alkaline; also help purify the blood and increase urine flow

radishes volatile oils help to stimulate digestion and bile production, even easing blocked bile flow

tarragon cleanses the kidneys and the gall bladder and has a mildly diuretic effect

vervaine commonly available as a tea, it is powerful enough to be used to help treat jaundice and an inflamed gallbladder

Below is a list of some of the most potent herbs and spices you can take to improve liver performance and to protect it from damage. They can be bought in either capsule or tincture form.

milk thistle The extract of this botanical remedy is called silymarin, and there is solid scientific evidence that it acts as a powerful liver healer. It can help to prevent, and reverse, liver damage by encouraging liver cells to repair and regenerate themselves. In Germany, the herb is a government endorsed supportive treatment for chronic liver inflammatory conditions. Milk thistle has also been found to reduce fatty degeneration of the liver and, in addition, prevents the entry of virus toxins and other toxic components, including drugs which can damage liver tissue. It can also act to reduce damage wrought by wild mushroom poisoning. Milk thistle contains a liver specific antioxidant which is a more powerful protector than vitamins E and C against damage to the liver. One of the key means by which silymarin improves detoxification is by preventing depletion of glutathione (see page 111). Sufficient levels of glutathione are critical for the liver to detoxify compounds, and milk thistle has been found to improve them by up to 35 per cent.

artichoke leaf This has a similar effect to milk thistle, and can promote regeneration and increase the blood flow to the liver. Artichoke leaf also helps to lower blood cholesterol levels. It is particularly useful for gall bladder disease.

dandelion root This is one of the oldest medicinal herbs, which is used to stimulate liver secretions and bile flow. As bile stimulating herbs can cause liver spasms if taken in large quantities, it is best taken with wild yam, which helps to prevent this problem.

green tea Contains compounds called flavonoid chatechins, which are strong antioxidants that have powerful liver protective effects. At levels of 10 cups a day, green tea has been shown to benefit cholesterol levels significantly while simultaneously improving other markers of liver health found in the blood.

turmeric This spice is commonly used in Middle Eastern and Asian cooking. It stimulates liver secretions and bile flow and also has powerful antioxidant properties. The main component, curcumin, improves detoxification in the liver. The whole plant is used by herbalists to help treat jaundice and liver disease.

yellow dock This is a blood cleanser and liver cleanser, which also stimulates the flow of bile. It helps to reduce inflamed tissues and eradicate excessive mucus production.

INSPIRATIONAL JUICES

Juices are frequently used as means of helping to cleanse the liver and to improve its functioning. The most commonly used juices for liver health are carrot and apple, but many other fruits, vegetables and herbs have beneficial effects. It is best to use organic produce, especially for the bases which form the bulk of the juice. Fortunately, organic carrots and apples are comparatively inexpensive.

● Tomatoes cleanse the blood and the liver. Mix tomato juice with celery, basil or beetroot.

● Orange, cabbage, papaya and pineapple juices help to improve digestion.

● Adding the zest of organic, non-waxed, citrus fruit (not grapefruit) to juices, and other dishes, is the best source of limonene, a potent trigger for the P450 enzyme system.

- Raspberries and grapes are superb for helping kidney function.
- Radish and watercress are high in sulphur. A good liver tonic uses 4 radishes, or 1 dandelion root, with 2 carrots and 1 apple.
- Beetroot stimulates liver drainage. Combine the root and leaves from half a raw beet with a couple of apples.
- Artichoke (globe) encourages bile flow and liver regeneration. Use the hearts of artichokes to add to vegetable juices such as tomato.
- Brassica vegetables such as broccoli, cabbage and cauliflower can be added to other juices. They taste best at a ratio of one part brassica vegetable to three parts other vegetables or fruit.
- Apples are one of the richest sources of quercitin, a valuable antioxidant, and they can be added to fruit or vegetable juices. Another very rich source is onions, particularly red onions, though they will be too strong for most people to add to juices. However, a little added to tomato juice can be quite delicious.
- Mangoes are rich in beta-carotene (300–3000 mcg per 100 g of flesh), as well as having good amounts of vitamins C and E. This makes them a good source of the antioxidant vitamins. All fruits and vegetables will be rich sources of antioxidants and drinking juices is the fastest way to assimilate them.

SUPPLEMENTING YOUR LIVER

In addition to the herbal supplements which are designed to support the liver, there are also a number of nutritional supplements (i.e. using vitamins and minerals and other food based compounds) which are also designed for this purpose. Here we will look at some of the most effective ones available.

vitamin C and glutathione Glutathione is found in virtually every living cell, and is particularly concentrated in the liver, kidneys, spleen, pancreas and eye cells. Early-evolution, one-celled plants probably used glutathione as an antioxidant to protect themselves from the harmful effects of oxygen. Animal and human cells use glutathione in much the same way. Glutathione also helps to detoxify many carbon compounds, and as we live in polluted environments with many carbon compounds and gases, this means of detoxification has added importance. Many toxic compounds, including heavy metals (see **Heavy Metals**, page 140), solvents and pesticides are fat-soluble, which makes them very difficult for the body to eliminate. The main route by which the body eliminates fat soluble compounds is in the bile, but 99 per cent of the bile is reabsorbed. This means that the fat-soluble compounds have to be made water soluble. And this is where glutathione comes in, allowing the compounds to be excreted in the urine. The elimination of these compounds, especially the heavy metals such as mercury and lead, is dependant upon there being enough glutathione in the body.

Glutathione is also needed for an important antioxidant enzyme. This combination of effects makes glutathione particularly valuable, and its deficiency can have far-reaching consequences on health. If we are exposed to large numbers of toxins, our reserves of this vital compound are depleted faster than they can be produced. In this way we are likely to become far more susceptible to toxicity-induced diseases, especially if Phase 1 is active and Phase 2 is working at below par.

Glutathione is available from the diet, as well as being synthesised in the body. It comes directly from fruit and vegetables and from cooked fish and meat. Gluthathione-rich sources are asparagus, avocado, cabbage, broccoli, Brussels sprouts, cauliflower and walnuts. It seems to be well absorbed in the intestines and is not broken down by digestion, making it instantly usable. While dietary glutathione is efficiently absorbed into the blood from foods, the same is probably not true for glutathione supplements. On the other hand, just 500 mg daily of vitamin C has been shown to raise blood glutathione levels significantly, by helping the body to synthesise it from other compounds. Vitamin C has even been shown to be effective in raising levels in people with an inherited deficiency of glutathione production. Vitamin C is also a powerful antioxidant and studies have shown that people with alcohol-induced liver disease had 50 per cent fewer blood markers of oxidation stress when they took 2.5 g for at least 14 days. Food sources of vitamin C are most fruits and vegetables, and their juices, and some of the best are citrus fruit, kiwis, strawberries, cabbages and broccoli. Though vitamin C seems to be the most effective, other compounds that help glutathione synthesis in the body are N-acetylcysteine (NAC), glycine and methionine.

glutamine This amino acid is not found in food, but is manu-factured in the body, and the area in which it is most concen-trated is the brain, where it is used as fuel. It has a number of helpful detoxification effects. First and foremost, it helps to get rid of toxic ammonia. It also increases the production of the liver's powerful detoxifier, glutathione (see above), and helps to prevent fatty liver degeneration. Glutamine is the primary fuel of the small intestines, and is important for both the colon and the pancreas. The latter produces digestive enzymes, so indi-rectly glutamine helps prevent damage to the digestive tract, where it can otherwise increase susceptibility to food allergies, which are a major factor in the accumulation of toxins. It helps to clear toxic wastes through the kidneys, and is also needed for the lymph system and the immune system to function properly (animal experiments have shown that deficiencies lead to an accumulation of bacteria in the lymph glands). Finally, by acting as a fuel for the brain, it helps curb cravings for cigarettes, alcohol, drugs and other stimulants, while at the same time helps to reduce some of the damage that these substances cause to the body. Useful doses are in the range of 5–10 g daily (though not taken all at once), and it is more cost effective to use the powder, which is more or less tasteless, in juices rather than take capsules. Despite its helpful effect on the liver and the kidneys, glutamine must not be taken if there is severe damage to either of these organs, or if you are pregnant or breast feeding.

lecithin This is the popular name for phosphatidyl choline, a form of fat called a phospholipid. Lecithin is found in cell membranes and helps fat soluble substances, including vitamins and hormones, to pass into and out of cells. It is because lecithin is a part of the structure of cells that it can help to regenerate damaged tissue, and it is particularly helpful for liver tissue, where it is more concentrated.

In studies, lecithin has been found to improve health in alcoholic liver disease and viral hepatitis, and because lecithin helps the transport of fat-soluble substances out of the cells, it is also likely to help speed up the removal of toxins from cells. Also, because lecithin is a fat emulsifier (it is often used in products such as ice cream, where it is used to mix together fats and water), it is immensely useful for helping people whose fat digestion capability is below par.

Lecithin can be bought either as capsules or granules. The latter are inexpensive and, as they have a pleasant taste, can be added to a variety of dishes; you can even eat them straight off the spoon. Since lecithin is a rich source of the B vitamins choline and inositol, the granules are also an economical way of supplementing them. Good food sources of lecithin include liver (though it is best to eat only organic in order to avoid pollutants), meat, fish, eggs, wheat, peanuts and soya.

cysteine This is a water-soluble sulphur amino acid which is found in wheatgerm, cottage cheese, yoghurt, turkey, duck and oats. It is able to help the body to process and render harmless chemicals as toxic as methyl isocyanat, which was involved in a huge number of deaths in Bhopal, India, in 1985. Cysteine with vitamin C can help to protect against the toxic effects of cigarette smoke and, to a degree, can also protect the lungs. It's derivative, N-acetyle cysteine (NAC), has been shown, in smokers and in non-smokers alike, to help liquefy mucus and loosen mucus plugs from the lungs, and has been used for asthma, bronchitis, cystic fibrosis and emphysema. However, do not supplement cysteine if you are an insulin dependant diabetic, as it supports insulin degeneration. The usual way to take cysteine for detoxification is to take it as N-acetyle cysteine, around 1 g daily.

taurine This is one of the sulphur containing amino acids, and is used for conjugation in the process of detoxification. It is also an antioxidant. Except in the case of babies, who cannot manufacture taurine (it is found in breast milk and must be added to formulas), it is made in the body from cysteine (see above). Supplementation is generally thought to be unnecessary, but it is not known if the natural amount made is enough for modern detoxification needs. Taurine deficient individuals may become very sensitive to aldehydes, chlorine, bleach and other similar compounds. Poor kidney function may result in taurine deficiency.

specific preparations There are some nutritional preparations (listed in **Resources**, page 171) which are specific formulations for liver support. These are useful for what are termed 'pathological detoxifiers'. This is when the P450 system is not synchronised correctly and Phase 1 is working faster than Phase 2, and they are designed to help to rectify this situation. These supplements variously combine taurine, glutamine and cysteine along with other free-form amino acids.

Liver support supplement programme

Diet always comes first when aiming to resolve any health problem. There is little point in taking copious amounts of supplements to help your liver to regenerate if you are still drinking excessive amounts of alcohol and eating few fruits and vegetables. Assuming that you have addressed your diet as summarised at the beginning of this chapter, and as covered in more detail in later chapters, I would suggest the following general liver support programme for most people. Follow it for at least three months.

- Drink 225 ml freshly made juice at least four times a week. Choose from the suggestions listed in **Inspirational Juices**, page 109. Include either carrot, apple or brassica vegetables in all the juices.

- Take a good quality multi-vitamin and mineral supplement daily. See **Resources**, page 171 for some suggested brands.

- Take 1–3 g daily of vitamin C in divided doses. Choose a non-acidic version, such as magnesium ascorbate, potassium ascorbate or calcium ascorbate. You can use powdered versions, and add them to juices or cereals if you do not like to take too many capsules.

- Take a herbal liver support supplement. The most effective

- is likely to be milk thistle, or a combination of milk thistle with other important herbs such as dandelion and artichoke.
- If you want even more liver protection, I would also add powdered L glutamine (1–2 teaspoons, 5–10 g) and a tablespoon of lecithin into your programme. Because these can be added to drinks and foods you do not have to pop too many capsules.
- An alternative to taking L-glutamine is to take one of the liver specific combination formulas listed in **Resources**, page 171.

THE CLAY CURE

Clay has been used, certainly since Biblical times, in external poultices to draw out impurities through the skin and to enhance healing of wounds and ulceration. Particular clays, with specific mineral make-ups, have been used for different purposes, and some are attributed greater healing powers than others. But did you know that clay can also be taken internally to enhance detoxification? I am not talking about clay dug up from the bottom of the garden pond, but of clay specifically prepared for the purpose.

Clay has a negative electrical attraction for particles that are positively charged, and so acts like a magnet to them. Most toxic poisons are positively charged, with the result that clay has great therapeutic value in detoxification. The large surface area of the clay molecules mean that they can pick up many times their weight in positively charged particles. According to a report by Robert T. Martin, a mineralogist at MIT in the US, 1 g of clay has a surface area of 800 square metres! Clay does not seem to have any chemical effect on the toxin particles, and 'the attraction is purely physical'. It is so powerful a detoxifier that clay has also been used in acute cases of poisoning to remove poison substances, such as arsenic, from the victims' system.

The most commonly available clay is green clay, though many others exist, including red, white, grey and yellow. Green clay is readily available from good quality health food shops, the most popular type being bentonite.

Clay must be taken in liquid form with water, otherwise it does not work quite so effectively, as tableting the clay changes the electrical properties. As you can imagine, clay tastes like – well, clay! It is an acquired taste. It is best to prepare the clay in advance, usually the night before, for use the following morning. Put a teaspoon of clay into half a glass of unboiled, filtered water. Do not leave a metallic spoon in contact with the clay mixture. Drink it in the morning, at least 15 minutes before eating, though an hour before is best (if you have forgotten to prepare it the previous night, you can still take it freshly made). A teaspoon daily is usually sufficient, as more may have the effect of obstructing the bowels. If it does cause constipation, drink the concoction slowly throughout the day instead of in one go. Because clay is so powerful, it is best, if you have recently been unwell or are in a very unfit state, to start the treatment slowly. Take a quarter teaspoon at first, and gradually build up the dose. In cases of diarrhoea, you may want to experiment with increasing the dose to 2 or even 3 teaspoons daily. Take the clay for three weeks initially, then rest for one week. After this take for one week, followed by a week-long rest, and continue in this way. It is generally not recommended to take clay until a course of medication has been finished, as it may adversely affect absorption of the drug you are taking.

Apart from promoting a general improvement in health as a result of improved elimination of toxins, taking clay, either orally or as topical poultices, can help conditions as diverse as stomach and duodenal ulcers, severe acne and rheumatic arthritis.

The Purest Drink of All?

To talk about detoxification without discussing water is equivalent to talking about gardening without thinking about rainfall. We all know that plants survive in desert conditions, but survive is the word – not thrive. And survival is tough.

In our damp climate, where water seems to be everywhere, we often fail to appreciate what a valuable commodity it is and instead take it for granted. The average person uses a massive 30 gallons of water daily for bathing, cooking, drinking and watering the garden.

Water is the second most important nutrient, after air, and we cannot function without it. To survive we cannot go for more than three days without water, but to thrive we need optimal amounts. Drinking sufficient water is not only essential medicine if you are feeling unwell or generally below par, it is also a basic requirement for maintaining excellent health if you are already lucky enough to possess it. Around 70 per cent of our bodies consist of water – ranging from 22 per cent of our seemingly solid bones to 92 per cent of our blood. Water is necessary for every body function – digestion, absorption, circulation, lubrication, regulation and, of course, elimination and detoxification, as it enables toxins to be transported away from cells for elimination through the kidneys. Many health problems can be partly attributed to insufficient water intake. If you suffer from aching joints, arthritis, headaches, migraines, blocked sinuses, dry skin, eczema, psoriasis, acne, constipation, diarrhoea, asthma or bronchitis you may need to drink more water. Even if you don't have any of these symptoms, you probably still need to drink more water, since the majority of us are in varying states of dehydration.

THE SOLUTION TO POLLUTION IS DILUTION

When the body is carrying an excess toxic load one of its solutions is to dilute the toxins by retaining water. Water is also the means by which toxins are flushed out of body tissues for excretion in the urine. Water is vital for detoxification.

During the Iranian revolution of 1979, the author of *Your Body's Many Cries for Water*, Dr F Batmangelidj, who was educated and trained in the UK, was imprisoned. During this time he acted as physician to his fellow prisoners. Lacking the necessary medicines, Dr Batmangelidj frequently relied upon water to treat his patients and he found that many conditions, such as peptic ulcers and bad backs, responded well. He came to the conclusion that many people suffer from chronic dehydration, induced by our modern lifestyle. Tea, coffee and colas have replaced water as a beverage, leading to, or exacerbating, diverse health problems. If the body is dehydrated, water will be allocated to vital functions such as heart and brain function. When dehydration occurs muscles and non-essential tissues are affected, leading to pain and other symptoms. By the time the sensation of thirst is felt, there is already dehydration throughout the body. I have seen many cases of chronic constipation, lower back pain and headaches resolved by the simple measure of eliminating dehydrating drinks from the diet and improving water intake.

DO YOU DRINK ENOUGH WATER?

You may think that you drink enough liquids already, but when we are talking about water we are not talking about strong tea, coffee, colas, cordials or alcohol. Any caffeine or alcohol containing drinks will ultimately be dehydrating as they cause a net loss of water from the body and this makes the job of detoxification harder. Sugary drinks, or those which are artificially sweetened, either cause increased thirst or play havoc with the body's chemistry, which in turn leads to an increased need for water.

At least 1.5 litres daily is needed for most people, and 2 litres daily is even better. If the weather is particularly hot or if you are breast feeding or doing a lot of manual work or exercise, you may need more than this. The only time when you need to be concerned about drinking this amount of water is if you have kidney damage, in which case talk to your doctor. If you suffer from prostate problems, drinking water is a part of the resolution to the problem, though you may want to avoid drinking in the evening to avoid the discomfort of being kept awake by your bladder.

When I talk about drinking water, I mean in its pure and unadulterated form, although there are ways that you can vary the experience if necessary. There are, for example, a variety of interesting herbal and fruit teas, such as red bush (rooibos) tea, lemon and ginger, mint and green tea, vervaine, camomile and blackcurrant, which can be drunk either hot or iced with fruit slices and mint leaves, sweetened with a little honey if you wish. You can also mix your water with freshly squeezed fruit juice (2/3 water to 1/3 juice) or flavour it with a small amount of blackcurrant or elderflower cordial made using fructose (fruit sugar available from health food shops) instead of sugar. Ring the changes by using sparkling water instead of still water. JUST DRINK WATER!

QUALITY AS WELL AS QUANTITY

We need water in copious quantities, but it is not just the amount that is critical, the quality is important too.

So is water the purest drink of all? It is an unfortunate reflection on our society that the three essentials for life – air, water and food – are treated in such a cavalier fashion with little regard to their quality. It may seem that we have any number of Government agencies to legislate for, and monitor, standards, but in reality we are paying a hefty price for the industrialisation of our society and the knock-on effect it has on our most basic requirements.

It is true that water quality in the West has improved to the extent that it no longer presents a serious danger to public health. By and large it is safe to drink, and we no longer have problems with water borne pathogens, such as those which cause typhoid or cholera. The problems we have now are more insidious and harder to measure in the short term. In the absence of health scares linked directly to water, it is fair to say that we have become complacent. And yet we have very real problems with our water quality right now. Our water is a repository for a myriad of chemicals that leach from industrial and agricultural sources. There is also concern about the levels of painkillers, antibiotics and hormones (from the Pill) that find their way into our water – in a large city such as London the water has been through 25 people before it gets to you! It is not only our reservoirs and wells which are contaminated, we are even managing to pollute the rain! A recent study found that much of Europe's water is rendered unfit to drink due to pesticide levels in rainwater running into the drinking water supply. European law has established certain acceptable levels of residues which are breached after heavy rain storms. The contamination seems to be greatest when the rainfall happens after a long dry spell. What is worrying about these chemicals is that a number of them have been linked to hormone disruption in humans as well as in animals. The potential effects of this include genital and fertility abnormalities and certain cancers, such as breast, ovarian, endometrial, testicular and prostate cancers.

As well as the problem of run-off from agricultural chemicals, we are also experiencing increasing acid rain. Gas-forming products from, for instance, car exhausts and aerosols, increase the deposition of sulphur dioxide, nitric oxide and ammonia, which is transported across continents in rainwater. Our environment is being radically transformed by the processes of industrialisation and convenience living.

Nitrates find their way into our drinking water by running off from artificial fertilisers. They break down in the stomach into nitrite, and then possibly into nitrosamines, compounds which are toxic and potentially carcinogenic. Nitrate also destroys vitamins A and E. Rural areas are particularly susceptible to this problem and EEC standards are regularly breached. Apart from eliminating nitrates from our drinking water, the most useful weapon we have against them is to make sure that we take in enough vitamin C, which helps to prevent the conversion of nitrates into nitrites and nitrosamines, from fruit and vegetables and, if necessary, from supplements.

In addition to the chemicals that run off from industrial processes, there is also the problem of heavy metals. Many of the conduits for water are still lead or copper, which can result in these two metals entering the water supply. There is no healthy level for lead, and while copper is a necessary mineral too much can be damaging to health. The pollutants all need to be handled by the human body, by our livers and kidneys, and detoxified. This places a strain on our already badly overworked organs and contributes to ill health.

IMPROVING YOUR WATER QUALITY

The problems with our water quality cannot necessarily be detected by taste, sight or smell, although over-chlorination produces cloudiness, as well as a strong smell, and if the water is foaming it may be a sign of bacterial contamination. If you are serious about following a detoxification programme, I would suggest that you need to be suspicious about the quality of your water supply and take steps to ensure that it is the best obtainable. Because we cannot see the contaminants it does not mean that they are not there, or that they are not harmful. A small number of people, who work at detoxing their system, never get completely well until they substitute mineral or distilled water for tap water.

Contact your local water board if you suspect that your water conduit is via lead pipes. Never use the water from the hot tap as it dissolves heavy metals far more readily than cold water does. Boiling tap water will reduce the risk of bacterial contamination if you suspect that this is a problem. If you use bottled water, check that the source of the water is of good quality. The regulations governing mineral water are stringent, though not as stringent as they are for tap water, so you are reliant upon good quality manufacturers. 'Spring' water is not covered by the same rules. It is quite possible for the manufacturers to use the equivalent of tap water and still call it spring water. It is also better to buy your water in glass bottles to avoid overexposure to pthalates from plastics.

As a minimum, I would suggest that you invest in a good quality water filter jug, of the type that is readily available from department stores and health food shops. Use the filtered water both for cooking, as well as for hot and cold drinks. Remember, however, that filters can become breeding grounds for bacteria, so regularly replacing the filter, and cleaning the filter housing, is essential. A good quality filter should eliminate, or greatly reduce, the levels of heavy metals such as lead, cadmium and mercury, it should reduce levels of fluoride and chlorine and remove any adverse taste, colour and odour in the water. If you want to go to the next level of convenience, though also of expense, you can buy plumbed in, activated carbon filters to use at your kitchen sink. These are effective at removing chlorine, heavy metals and many organic compounds. However, they may not be good at eliminating nitrates, and cannot be relied upon to remove bacterial contaminants.

You can also buy a more sophisticated type of filter, called a reverse osmosis system, which forces water under pressure through a semi-permeable membrane. It is fairly effective and inexpensive to run, but the storage tank takes up a lot of space and it needs regular maintenance. There are also questions as to whether the synthetic membranes themselves add to chemical contamination of the water, due to the high pressures used.

Distillation is one of the most efficient means of removing contaminants because it evaporates the water for collection in a jug and very few contaminants are carried over in this way. This is the most expensive system available. As all the minerals which are present in water are also removed, some people question whether this is desirable, as it has been shown that minerals in water can have various health benefits. However, another school of thought suggests that if the person is eating a diet which is high in mineral-rich foods, such as fruit, vegetables, legumes, nuts, seeds, grains and small amounts of dairy produce and meat, minerals from water are not necessary.

A CLEANSER AND A HEALER

Water is a balm for our bodies in many other ways. Water therapies abound, and even the least health-aware person will understand the healing power of a cold compress for a headache, an ice pack for a swelling or a hot bath to ease muscle tension. We are naturally drawn to water and its healing properties. An effective remedy for bronchial or asthmatic patients is to spend time by the sea, to benefit from the effect that the water has by charging the air with healing negative ions. Steam inhalations are the best way to relieve catarrh, and a herbal or sea salt bath is one of the best ways of relaxing. A warm shower, alternating with cold blasts of water, is a truly invigorating way of setting yourself up for the day (it feels much better than it sounds, and you can slowly turn the mixer tap on to the cold setting instead of jolting yourself into the stratosphere!). Plunging your hands or feet into alternating hot and cold tubs of water will stimulate all the acupuncture points which begin and end at the extremities (though never make the water hot enough to burn you). Hydrotherapy is one of the cheapest, most readily available and useful means of healing our bodies. The first place to start is by drinking more water, but don't forget about all the other uses for water.

. . . .

Clean Up Your Act

. . . .

So far I have concentrated on the positive ways diet can encourage detoxification through increasing the amount of fruit and vegetables we eat daily, drinking more water and adding more health-giving herbs to our cooking. This is the way I prefer to work, since it encourages a more positive outlook when changing eating and exercise habits. If you are doing more of what is good for you, there is a greater chance that you are crowding out what does not work for you.

Nevertheless, there comes a point where we really do need to address our residual habits and living conditions. And this is what this chapter is all about. By eating more healthily you will be supporting your liver and other detoxification organs, but if you continue to expose yourself to a wide range of pollutants, your body will inevitably find it hard to keep up with processing toxins. A sample taken from an average Egyptian mummy has virtually no chemicals in the tissues (apart from those used for embalming), whereas one taken from someone today contains hundreds of different foreign chemicals.

This chapter focuses on the most important environmental and dietary sources of pollutants, and the best ways of eliminating them from your body, and your life.

HOME SICK?

To recap, we are exposed to a potential 60,000 chemicals from our environment and food on a regular basis, and 400 of these circulate in the average home. By reducing our exposure to as many of these as possible we will lighten the load that our liver has to deal with.

Most of us spend 80–90 per cent of our time indoors, where the levels of some pollutant gases are up to ten times higher than those recorded outside. This, worryingly, leads to a 'cocktail effect' that is likely to be even more damaging. Gas cookers, coal and wood fires, and gas and paraffin heaters all burn up fresh air and produce toxic gases such as carbon monoxide. Synthetic furnishings and cleaning products all contribute to the indoor pollution, as do building materials such as chipboard and vinyl flooring, which also contain glues and can give off formaldehyde, a pollutant to which a significant number of people are sensitive in concentrations as low as one part per million. If you have a garage attached to your house, you can have up to 80 per cent more benzene in your home than if you share your home with a heavy smoker (which, in any case, can take you above the maximum level recommended for outdoors). Alongside these hazards are 'biological' pollutants such as house dust mites and moulds, and the danger of being unfortunate enough to live in a high radon area – 2,000 people a year die from radon-induced lung cancer (for details about having your house tested for radon by your local authority, see **Resources**).

Even buying beauty products can be hazardous. Remember the days when it was impossible to walk through a department store without being assaulted by a coiffured beautician spraying you with scent? Without anyone noticing they have been disappearing, and now you have to ask before you get a whiff as the manufacturers now recognise the potential problem. More than 9,000 chemicals are licensed for use in cosmetics alone. One of the most commonly used, to produce foam and bubbles in bath and hair products, is SLS (sodium laureth sulfate), which is used in industry because it is so efficient at stripping grease and oil off surfaces such as garage floors. SLS can also react with other chemicals, leading to dioxin absorption through the skin. It is usually used in concentrations of between 10–30 per cent but can be used at levels of up to 50 per cent. Tests have shown that concentrations over 15 per cent can cause serious skin irritation. Products also often use propylene glycol, otherwise known as anti-freeze, and this has been linked to kidney and liver damage.

AVOIDING CHEMICALS

As with eating habits, it takes time to make changes in your buying habits for household products and toiletries, to become aware of suppliers of chemical-free alternatives. Make a pact with yourself, however, that you will invest the time that is needed. The following tips and ideas should help you in your quest to reduce your exposure to unnecessary chemicals.

- **Buy organic food whenever possible** You can keep the cost of your shopping basket down by preparing more meals from scratch, and relying less upon convenience foods, organic or otherwise. In this way you can work with what is in season and reasonably priced. You will find that items such as beans, pulses and grains are all inexpensive and make superb bases for a wide range of dishes. Vegetables and fruits in season can be bought in bulk and frozen, and certain vegetables, such as root vegetables, are always reasonable.

- **Wash all produce thoroughly** Non-organic produce is likely to have some residues of farming chemicals on the surface (plus more, unfortunately, within). A little vinegar in water will help to strip alkaline pesticides from fruits and vegetables, and bicarbonate of soda will strip acid residues. Use two bowls with the two compounds in them and soak/wash your fruit and vegetables in each bowl in turn. If necessary, peel the produce. It is as well to wash both non-organic and organic produce.

- **Restrict your dependence on foods in cans or cartons** While there are some staples that can be very useful as standbys, if you find that you are opening cans on a daily basis it is best to cut down. The thin plastic coating which lines the cans is likely to leach chemicals into the food.

- **Avoid using plastics in food preparation** This means getting rid of clingfilm and plastic food storage containers. Store food in ceramic or glass containers, and use grease-proof paper instead of clingfilm to cover dishes (you can always use clingfilm or foil to seal it over the top of the greaseproof paper).

- **Use porcelain, glass or stainless steel cookware in preference to other types** Even non-stick pans may leach the metal fluoride into food.

- **Use a water filter to remove chlorine, or buy mineral water** (preferably in glass bottles) or distil your water (see The Purest Drink of All?, page 118).

- **Use personal care products that are based on natural ingredients** If these ingredients are used in food which you are happy to eat you can be happy about putting them on your skin and in your bath (see Resources, page 176).

- **Keep chemicals in and around your house, garden and car to a minimum** Avoid using pesticides, wood treatments, or hair lice products (you can use herbal lice products instead, or use the wet combing method described in leaflets available from all pharmacies). Also eliminate all products in aerosol cans.

- **Pay particular attention to your bedroom** as you spend over a third of your life there. Make sure that fabrics

are not treated with chemicals, that mattresses and pillows
do not harbour moulds, and think about choosing wooden
flooring in preference to carpet. Do not bring dry-cleaned
clothes into your room and air them first.

- **Use natural detergents** for washing dishes, clothes and as
  body soaps.
- **Use unbleached alternatives** for products such as
  lavatory paper, coffee filters (which are hopefully now
  redundant anyway!), kitchen paper and tampons, all of
  which are now readily available from supermarkets, health
  food shops and by mail order.
- **Remove synthetic materials from home and workplace
  as far as you are able** This includes removing plastics,
  vinyls, foam rubber and chipboard, toxic cleaning chemicals and polishes, synthetic soaps, detergents and perfumed
  products. Use non-toxic paints and varnishes, unperfumed
  detergents, natural soaps and shampoos. Use untreated
  cotton for bedding or clothing (which is much more
  attractive anyway). Avoid dry cleaning, detergents or fabrics which contain formaldehyde.
- **Open windows regularly** on opposite sides of the house
  to create cross-ventilation and to help eliminate chemical
  build-up.
- **Invest in low light houseplants**, such as bamboo, ferns,
  palms and chrysanthemums as they reduce levels of chemicals, in particular formaldehyde (one plant per 100 square
  feet is recommended). Surprisingly tea bags scattered
  around rooms have been shown to reduce formaldehyde
  levels by 60 per cent to 90 per cent as the tannin in the tea
  helps the leaves absorb it.

Suppliers of chemical-free products are listed in **Resources**, page
171.

Use these alternatives to get chemicals out of your life

- filtered water instead of tap water
- porcelain or glass food storage containers
- stainless steel, porcelain or glass cookware
- greaseproof paper (secure with clingfilm or foil on the outside if necessary)
- glass bottles instead of plastic
- foods packaged in glass instead of in plastic lined cartons or tins
- organic foods and drinks
- unbleached paper and sanitary products
- fluoride-free toothpaste
- shampoos and bath products that exclude sodium lauryl sulfate, sodium laureth sulfate and propylene glycol
- mix your own aromatherapy scents instead of using commercially produced perfume
- swap your air freshener for a bowl of essential oils
- detergent and chlorine-free washing-up liquid and soap powders
- use baking soda instead of kitchen surface, oven and lavatory cleaners
- use herbal head lice products (or use the wet combing method)
- choose pump action toiletries and cleaning products instead of aerosol cans
- use olive oil instead of shoe polish – it adds life to leather
- unbleached cotton products
- fabrics that can be washed instead of dry cleaned
- use only natural building materials in the home (instead of foam, chipboard, etc), and ideally have hard flooring (stone, wood) and wet-mop regularly
- protective mattress and pillowcase covers

- use water-based paints or low VOC paints instead of gloss. Store surplus paints, paint strippers, etc, outside
- use electric instead of gas — gas flames should be blue (yellow flames indicate carbon monoxide)

FEARSOME FATS?

It is not uncommon for a person on a typical SAD (Standard American Diet — which is also typical of many other Western countries such as the UK) to take in more fat than their liver can cope with efficiently. Apart from the metabolic stress that this puts on the liver, it also presents a problem because chemicals, many of them toxic, accumulate in fats. In this way, dietary fats can add to the burden of excess toxins. Body fat cells are also repositories of these chemicals. It is highly desirable to make sure that the fats and fatty foods you eat, such as dairy produce and meats, are organic. By the same token, vegetables and fruits which have been sprayed with fat soluble pesticides are best avoided, and organic choices made, even if they are a little less evenly grown and a little more expensive.

Fat soluble toxins pose another worrying problem. The most subtle, and therefore the most dangerous, impact on our body chemistry comes from substances which resemble our own hormones. In this way they go unnoticed in the short term, but have a sneaky effect on our health in the long term. They mimic our own natural hormones, blocking the action of the natural hormones, and therefore affecting their necessary functions. These Trojan horses are called xenohormones, which are a by-product of agricultural, pharmaceutical and manufacturing processes. In particular, the manufacture of plastics, that 20th century wonder, is one of the most common household sources of these xenohormones. Like our own hormones, these are fat soluble, and come in to the food supply through fats in the diet.

The agri-chemicals used on animal feeds, grasses and grains concentrate in animal fats such as the meat and dairy produce we eat. They are also present in sprays that are used in the production of fruits and vegetables. We also consume them from foods which have been wrapped in plastic bags, clingfilm and plastic containers. These xenohormones are implicated in the huge increase in breast, ovarian, womb, prostate and testicular cancers.

Fats of any kind, if they go rancid or are processed or overheated, can contribute to fatty degeneration problems (such as cholesterol build up in arteries) by creating damaging free radicals that damage body tissues and cholesterol. This means that it is best to use very fresh oils for dressing salads, and for other culinary uses. Oils such as walnut oil, sesame oil, flax oil and safflower oil can be highly beneficial, but only if they are fresh. They are beneficial because they form a part of the healthy structure of cell walls, including the liver, and are used to make hormones. These oils need to be bought in small, light-proof bottles, must be used by the sell by date, and kept in the fridge once opened. The fat that is least likely to create problems of rancidity, that is also of benefit to your liver, is olive oil. You can use it for cooking (though do not allow it to smoke at very high temperatures), you can spread it on your bread, you can add it to salads. Avocados and very fresh nuts and seeds (sunflower, pumpkin, flax, sesame) are other excellent sources of beneficial fats. You can also use nut butters such as almond nut butter, cashew nut butter, sesame seed butter or tahini as spreads (but, again, keep them in the fridge once opened).

Oily fish are another superb source of the beneficial fats that we use to build cells and brain tissue, and they are also important in promoting a healthy heart and in reducing inflammatory problems such as arthritis. The fats in oily fish are also important in the fight against breast cancer, though there is considerable

concern that they are also sources of dioxin and mercury contamination. On balance, however, I think the benefits of the fish
oils outweigh the damage that the toxins they carry are likely to
do and, if the diet is generally healthy, there is an increased ability to eliminate the mercury (though dioxins are more difficult
to get rid of). It helps, of course, if you are keeping your exposure to other chemical pollutant sources low (dairy products are
also a major source of dioxin exposure).

The oils that tend to be available cheaply in bulk, such as
sunflower, corn and soya, have usually been extracted using
chemical solvents or at high temperatures sufficient to damage
the fats. As a result, I would avoid them and substitute organic
extra-virgin olive oil or some other delicious oil such as walnut
or flax. Margarines are also highly processed and are frequently
high in hydrogenated fats, so I would generally avoid these too.
Instead you can use a number of other spreads on your bread,
including olive oil, flax oil, nut butters, tahini, hummus and
various vegetable pâtés and tapenadas.

ALCOHOL – LIVER ENEMY No. I

Alcohol is insidious because it exerts its toxic effect on the
body in a variety of ways. It interrupts a number of essential
chemical processes in the body, such as those that allow the
healthy fats to convert into hormones and into inflammation
regulating substances. It is because of this that alcohol is
implicated in, or at least contributes to, a number of different
inflammatory problems. Alcohol also has a particularly negative
effect on the liver enzymes that are responsible for a significant
amount of the body's detoxification. By exerting this effect, it
acts as a sort of super-toxin, reducing the ability of the detoxification enzyme system to deal with other toxins, thus letting
them get more of a foothold than they would otherwise do. This

is why the packaging of various medicines carries the advice to avoid alcohol.

Alcohol is easily absorbed and is taken to the liver for disarming. Getting tipsy is a direct consequence of exceeding your liver's immediate ability to detoxify the alcohol. People have different rates at which they deal with alcohol, though, generally speaking, men's livers process alcohol more efficiently than women's do, simply because they are larger. The zinc dependent enzyme, alcohol dehydrogenase, is the first step in dealing with alcohol. At the end of Phase 1 detoxification, the chemical left is acetaldehyde, which often causes worse symptoms than the alcohol itself – hence the hangover (a combination of acetaldehyde and dehydration).

Alcohol causes 80 per cent of all liver disease in Western countries. It directly damages the liver and increases the amount of fatty deposits in the organ. The accepted view is that women have the capacity to cope with one measure of alcohol daily, and that men can deal with two. This does not mean that if you have not had a drink for several days you can catch up by having several in one go – your liver can still only deal with a certain amount in a 24-hour period. Research has suggested that one or two measures of alcohol daily may contribute to a reduced risk of heart disease. This may be true for men, and for women past the age of menopause, but in women of a reproductive age alcohol can increase oestrogen to levels that can lead to hormone imbalance problems. The latest research suggests that one or two measures a week have health benefits, which are not improved by drinking one to two measures a day (as was previously thought).

It is generally believed that wine provides greater health benefits than other forms of alcohol. Beer, for example, is high in yeasts which, in susceptible people, can encourage unfriendly bowel bacteria to proliferate. Certainly red wine has antioxidants in it, called proanthocyanidins, which are highly protective against a number of diseases. However, red wine also contains high levels of histamines, which can trigger allergic reactions in susceptible people. If you find that red wine makes you flushed and headachy, it might be an idea to switch to white wine or spirits, though it would be better to cut out alcohol altogether for a while to give your system a rest, and then to drink only in moderation. And if the antioxidants are your excuse for drinking red wine, just remember you can get a similar amount from red grape juice!

If you want to continue to enjoy an occasional drink, it can only help if you make your choice from some of the excellent organic wines that are now available. L-Glutamine (discussed in **Nature's Helping Hand**, page 106) can be helpful in reducing alcohol cravings. There are also other supplements that are useful as well – the antioxidants, such as vitamins C and E, or N-acetyle cysteine (also discussed previously) can help to protect against some of the liver damage from alcohol.

COFFEE CRAVINGS

Coffee raises levels of an enzyme called alanine aminotransferase, high levels of which are an indication of liver damage. Coffee has also been shown to raise levels of LDL (bad) cholesterol and blood fats, which can also suggest an effect on the liver. Interestingly, this effect is less marked with filter coffee as opposed to cafetière coffee. So if you absolutely cannot give up your one essential cup of morning coffee, you would be better off having organic filter coffee. If you use instant coffee, make sure it is organic as the process of drying the coffee uses a number of different chemicals that your body can do without.

If you have severe caffeine intolerance, and even a small amount keeps you awake at night, there is a good chance that your Phase 1 detoxification is impaired. This may be masked by heavy coffee or tea use, so if, after avoiding caffeine for a couple of weeks, you find that you have a strong rebound reaction, it may be a good idea to look at rebalancing your Phase 1 and 2 systems (see page 28).

Decaffeinated coffee is not the solution either, because although the caffeine has been removed, the two other members of the methylxanthine group of chemicals – theophillyne and theobromine – remain.

One of the best alternatives to coffee is dandelion coffee, because dandelion is supportive of liver health. However, when commercially made, it tends to contain a lot of lactose (milk sugar), so if you are intolerant to lactose you may need to give it a miss. Other options include chicory, barley and acorn coffees, all of which are delicious, and readily available from health food shops.

Giving up coffee can result in a number of unpleasant side effects. As your liver throws off accumulated toxins, you go through a drug withdrawal stage, which brings the stress hormone adrenaline into play. Short-term effects can include sweats, headaches, a metallic taste in your mouth, cloudy urine, constipation and blurred vision. None of these symptoms should last for more than four or five days, however, and when you get clear of this stage you will feel in much better shape than when you were drinking coffee.

THE DEMON WEED

If you smoke, or live or work in a smoky atmosphere, this is one of the first things that needs to be addressed on your detox programme. The 2,000 chemicals found in cigarette smoke are some of the hardest for your body to deal with. Nicotine is only the tip of the iceberg. The nicotine, tar and the other substances in cigarette smoke, including the toxic compounds cadmium, arsenic, cyanide, nitrosamines and sometimes DDT, have to be dealt with by the liver. As it deals with the compounds by hydroxylation, more toxic compounds are produced which directly damage the liver. Additionally, carbon monoxide binds insolubly with haemoglobin in red blood cells, stopping them from carrying oxygen, and it takes 120 days for the lifeless blood cell to be broken down and eventually replaced. This leads to a variety of circulatory problems. There is no easy way to say this, other than, if you smoke – give it up now!

If you find you can't resist the craving for nicotine, try drinking a ¼ cup of lobelia tea or taking 10–20 drops of the herbal tincture several times a day when the craving strikes. This is thought to help because the chemical lobeline, found in lobelia, closely resembles nicotine. Regular consumption of oats has also been shown to curb the need for cigarettes, which may be due to their sedative properties, as has taking L-glutamine. Taking the mineral chromium can help to stabilise blood sugar levels, which also may make giving up the weed a little more easy. If you continue to smoke, it is beneficial to take an antioxidant supplement, along with eating a lot of fruit and vegetables, to compensate for some of the damage that smoking causes.

DRUGS – MEDICINAL OR OTHERWISE

Coffee, alcohol, sugar and cigarettes can all be classified as drugs when you think about their addictive nature and the problems that most people have in giving them up! All other drugs, including over-the-counter (OTC) drugs, prescribed medication and recreational drugs, also have an effect on the liver. As it happens, many of them are only activated when they are processed via the liver. Addiction to OTC drugs in particular is becoming an increasing problem. Every year in the UK we spend £205 million on painkillers, £251 million on cold and cough remedies and £129 million on remedies for digestive disorders. And yet addressing diet and lifestyle is the most effective way of eliminating painful conditions such as headaches, some forms of arthritis and digestive problems such as constipation and diarrhoea. Improved diet also helps boost the immune system, enabling you to ward off colds and coughs.

If you find that you are using OTC drugs on a regular basis, this is something you can address without your doctor's input, and by following a detox programme you may find that the symptoms for which you were taking medication are relieved anyway.

If you are on prescribed medication, you can talk to your doctor about the possibility of reducing your dose if you begin to feel better when following a healthy eating plan. (You must not, however, stop prescribed medication without consulting your doctor.) It is particularly important to look out for the problems of multiple medication and the side effects that can result from this. Multiple medication tends to be a particular problem for older people who have had a number of drugs prescribed for a variety of reasons. It is not uncommon for side effects to the drugs, such as dizziness or constipation, to be treated by prescribing yet more medication!

If the drugs you prefer are recreational, then no matter what you have been told, or choose to believe, for example that marijuana is less damaging than tobacco, it is still the case that the chemicals affect the liver adversely and, even more worryingly, damage brain cells. If you are on a serious detoxification programme there is really no place on it for recreational drugs.

Various highly effective natural methods have been used to alleviate drug withdrawal in place of, for instance, the methadone that is used for heroin withdrawal. These methods entail going 'cold turkey'. While doing so, however, the person participates in an intensive programme that involves going on runs to sweat out as much of the drugs as possible through the pores, and taking several saunas a day for the same reason. Very high doses (several grams) of niacin, a form of vitamin B3 which causes flushing and sweating, are also given. Other supplements, such as spirulina and chlorella, have also been shown to alleviate drug withdrawal symptoms, L-glutamine can help to reduce cravings, and the amino acid glycine is good for assisting detox-ification of drugs and toxic chemicals. However, none of these supplements should be taken for drug withdrawal without pro-fessional supervision.

HEAVY METALS

We are not talking about rock 'n' roll here! These heavy metal compounds cause serious health problems for many people. Like many other pollutants, however, they are invisible and so are not taken very seriously. And yet recent Government statistics have shown that one in ten children in the UK is affected by lead lev-els which are sufficient to impair IQ. Lead poisoning is thought to have been a major factor in the demise of the Roman Empire, and if we are not careful we may go the same way! Lead toxic-ity usually results from old water piping, but it can also be absorbed from pollution, hair dye and even by children chewing old paintwork.

The main heavy metals we need to concern ourselves with are lead, cadmium, aluminium, mercury and, occasionally, arsenic. Copper is another metal which is a necessary nutrient, and dietary levels are often low. However, since we frequently rely on copper water piping it is not unusual to find that some individuals have adversely high levels, especially in soft water areas. Heavy metal toxicity is a major problem for pregnant women and can significantly affect the health of foetuses, resulting in low birth weights and small head circumferences. The main risk of this comes from cadmium from cigarette smoke, but other heavy metals are involved as well.

These heavy metals, along with a number of other factors such as food contaminants, alcohol and caffeine, are also termed anti-nutrients. This is because they can seriously interfere with the uptake of essential nutrients such as zinc, iron and B-vitamins from food. High blood levels, for instance of copper, resulting from taking the Pill or HRT, can result in a low zinc status. Equally, it is a waste of time drinking a cup of coffee after a meal, or with your vitamin and mineral supplements, because it will reduce the overall uptake of nutrients by around 25 per cent.

If you suspect that you may have high heavy metal levels in your body, the easiest way to check this is by a simple Hair Mineral Analysis test (see page 39).

The ways that we can reduce levels of toxic heavy metals are by:

- Avoiding sources of the heavy metals, for instance filtering your drinking water, being cautious about which cookware you use, checking your water conduit pipes and avoiding regular contact with cigarette smoke. It is even worth getting everyone to remove their shoes when they come in the house. Dust traipsed in from outside is one of the highest sources of low-level chronic lead exposure inside the house (which builds up) because old lead, from traffic fuel and other pollution, persists in the soil.
- Balancing your mineral levels, so that you have a healthy supply of those which are antagonistic to the heavy metals (i.e. help to stop you absorbing them). For instance, the mineral zinc is antagonistic to lead.
- Eating foods, and possibly taking supplements, which help to eliminate accumulated stores of heavy metals.

The foods that have the strongest potential to help detoxify heavy metals are pectin fibre, alginic acid in seaweeds and the 'green' foods spirulina and chlorella. Pectin fibre, found in apples, bananas and pears, is a strong eliminator of heavy metals and is readily available as a powdered fibre to sprinkle on foods. Seaweeds are easy to incorporate into your diet once you put your mind to it. The most straightforward way is to fill up a pepper mill with seaweed granules, which are available from health food shops, and to use this as a delicious condiment on soups, salads and any other savoury dish. You can also buy seaweed flakes to sprinkle on foods. Other seaweeds, such as nori and wakame, can be variously toasted and sprinkled on foods, or soaked and shredded and added to soups and stews. Spirulina and chlorella are available as tablets or in powdered form and are great to add to smoothies – creating your own green drinks

Heavy Metal	Sources
Lead	Lead water pipes (pre-1948 houses), traffic pollution (improved since lead-free petrol), cigarettes, old paintwork, lead toys, pencils, hair dyes, industry (e.g. car manufacturing)
Cadmium	cigarette smoke, refined and canned foods, detergents, fertilisers, new carpets
Aluminium	cookware and foil, antiperspirants, antacids, toothpaste, some table salts and processed cheese, cigarette filters

is great fun and names such as Green Dragon, Green Power and Green Machine spring to mind. Other foods with strong heavy metal detoxifying capabilities include alfalfa, mung beans, other beans and peas, lentils and beansprouts. Of all these, alfalfa sprouts are the nutritional leaders and are superb at enhancing detoxification.

The most potent all-round detoxifying nutrient is vitamin C (1–3 g daily), as it is able to 'escort' most of the heavy metals out of the body, and the most potent vitamin C formulations are those that come with bioflavonoids. The minerals selenium (100–200 mcg daily), magnesium (500 mg daily) and calcium (500 mg daily) are also virtually universal detoxifyers.

Check the chart below for sources of heavy metals and for a list of the nutrients that can help to detoxify them.

Affects	To detox
nervous system impairs IQ and bone health impairs absorption of zinc	calcium, zinc (which displaces lead), vit C, B1 & B6 (remove lead from the brain), pectin, alginic acid
high blood pressure bone health damages kidneys and nerves respiratory system	vit C, A & E, zinc, calcium, selenium, pectin, alginic acid, onion, garlic, leeks
may be implicated in Alzheimer's disease and dyslexia	calcium, zinc, magnesium, manganese, vit B6, silicon (herb horsetail)

Heavy Metal	Sources
Mercury	amalgam fillings, tuna and other large fish, fungicides and pesticides, some paints
Copper	copper water pipes, female hormone medication, i.e. HRT and the Pill, raises blood copper levels
Arsenic	some table salts, some beers and wines, some pesticides (used in cereal growing), dyes and paints, water in some developing countries
Fluoride	toothpastes and other oral hygiene products using sodium fluoride, fluoridated water, non-stick pans

Affects	To detox
brain function damages kidneys and liver, and possibly implicated in multiple sclerosis	selenium, eggs, onions, leeks, vit C, calcium, lecithin protects brain zinc, pectin,alginic acid
main signs are those of zinc and iron imbalance	zinc, iron, eggs, onions, garlic, leeks
respiratory system, liver, kidneys, implicated in skin cancer arsenate is quite well handled human body, but arsenite accumulates in vital organs organs	selenium, vits A, C, E, pectin, alginic acid
fluorosis (brown mottling of the teeth), thyroid problems, osteoporosis, immunity (possibly some cancers)	calcium fluoride does not have the damaging impact of sodium fluoride

Part Four

MORE DETOX

TOOLS

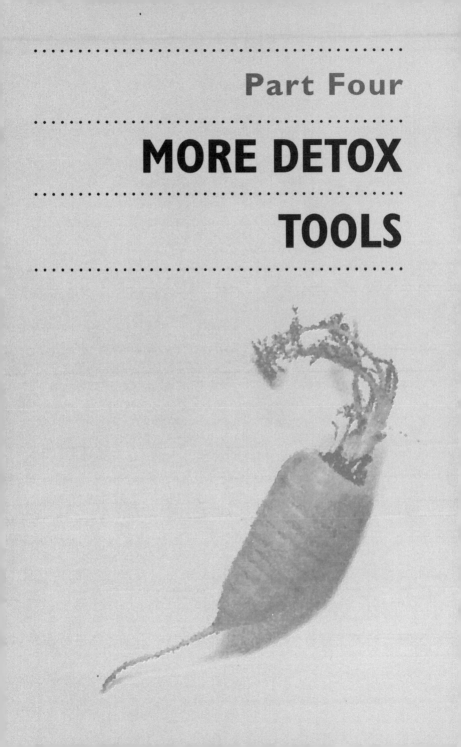

CHAPTER TEN

When Less
May be More

As with any approach to health, there are degrees of involvement that will suit some people and not others. The detox programmes we have discussed, and the rationales behind them, will suit the majority of people and the majority of complaints. However, there will always be some people who have intractable health problems that need a more intensive approach. Other possible therapeutic approaches to detoxing include fasting (when less may indeed be more), the liver and gall bladder flush, and enemas and colonic irrigation, all of which we will look at briefly here.

Whilst all these options have a place in health management, it is important not to start relying upon them. An occasional purge can never be a substitute for a healthy lifestyle. Your prime task is to master the basics of good nutrition, eating a balanced diet that suits your constitution and avoids pollutants and anti-nutrients. Once you have got the basics right, however, you may want to investigate some of the other methods that have been used by natural therapists for many years to improve health.

FASTING

Fasting has been used throughout the centuries as a means of restoring health and is one of the oldest known therapies. Indeed, it is usual for us to go off food when we are unwell, and while adults may override this urge in the mistaken belief that they need to eat to keep their strength up, babies, children and animals, who are more in touch with this natural response, will usually refuse food. The physical explanation for this is pretty straightforward. As the digestion and metabolism of food, and the subsequent need to detoxify waste products, is such an energy intensive process, the body's energy is naturally diverted towards healing by avoiding food for a while.

Fasting is the speediest means to increase elimination of wastes and stored toxins. However, it can be dangerous for some people, and needs to be conducted properly. Strictly speaking, fasting means abstaining totally from all food and drink, apart from water, for a specific period of time. It should never be undertaken without proper medical supervision, and caution should be exercised by those with a diagnosed medical condition. Diabetics, for example, may find that their blood sugar levels drop too low, too quickly, producing a diabetic coma. Serious kidney disease is another instance where fasting can be harmful if it is not supervised, and it should never be under taken by those who are severely underweight. It is also inappropriate to fast when you are pregnant or breast feeding. This is because you need to maintain a basic level of nutrient intake, plus the effects of liberating toxins into your system when nurturing a baby are likely to be detrimental. In addition, fasting is usually unsuitable for people who have excessive amounts of toxicity, as the reaction when stored toxins are liberated into the system can be very unpleasant, resulting in a serious exacerbation of symptoms and many undesirable new ones. It has also been found that people who 30 or 40 years ago took drugs such as LSD have had hallucinogenic experiences after going on a strict detoxification as drug residues are liberated from the liver.

On the positive side, however, fasting, especially combined with other therapies, has been described as 'awakening the physician within'. It can enhance healing potential as it allows both the mind and the body the time, space and physiological rest necessary to allow normalisation, harmony and recovery.

If you are planning to go on a fast, there are certain basic rules that you need to follow:

- Do not indulge in a fast at home of longer than two or three days.
- For a longer fast you must be under strict medical supervision, preferably in an inpatient facility or spa.
- During even a short fast of one day, you must drink copious amounts of water – at least one 225ml glass every half hour during waking hours. Water is needed to stay hydrated and to flush out the toxins that are released.
- Do not do any strenuous physical activity during a fast. For this reason it is best to undertake a fast when not at work. You may feel light-headed during a fast and driving or operating machinery is a bad idea.
- Rest is an important part of the fasting and detoxification ritual. You may feel fine, but it is still wise to take an afternoon nap, and to observe sensible sleeping hours at night. The more rest you have, the better the results, as energy can be focused on the healing process of detoxification.
- Stay warm, by wearing layers of clothing, as body temperature usually drops during a fast. Blood pressure, pulse and respiration rates may also drop, as your metabolic rate slows.
- Breaking a fast needs to be done sensitively. There is no point in going straight back into eating a heavy meal. It is best to ease slowly back into normal eating by making the first couple of meals fruit and vegetable based, and not overeating. It is also a good idea to chew food thoroughly, to eat food at room temperature, and to avoid caffeine and alcohol.

● If you need to take drugs for any reason, do not fast.

● The best fast for most people, which is usually just as effective as the more rigorous classical fast, is the modified fast, as described in the Three-day Intensive Detox, page 77.

● You must not even think about fasting if you have a tendency towards eating disorders. It is not sensible to focus on fasting if you are already battling with problems of bingeing or anorexia. If this is the case, you must sort your body chemistry out with sensible, healthy eating, and seek help with counselling.

● Do not take a sauna during a water fast (it is fine to do so during a modified fast such as the Three-day Intensive Detox).

● Do not take any supplemented nutrients during a water fast.

ONE-DAY JUICE FAST

An easier option than the full-blown water fast, is the one-day juice fast. Here the rules are pretty much the same, except that you can drink any amount of freshly made organic fruit or vegetable juice (see page 109 for some ideas) and herbal or fruit teas, just so long as you maintain your water intake as well. Following a one-day juice fast each week is of tremendous benefit, as it allows your body to throw off accumulated toxins before they have the chance to do too much damage to body organs. There is no great benefit, however, in doing it more frequently than this, as the body needs the nourishment, energy and building blocks that come from a healthy eating plan.

As with a water fast, you should not embark on a juice fast if you have a diagnosed medical condition. Indeed, the same cautions and rules apply here as well, plus the following specific ones too:

- Do not take vitamin and mineral supplements during a one-day juice fast as this gives your body more work to do. In any case, they work best within the context of eating proper meals.

- Before going on a one-day juice fast, prepare yourself by keeping your diet as simple as possible on the previous day. Eat more fresh fruit and vegetables, whole grains, sprouted seeds and beans, and avoid alcohol, caffeine and dairy products.

- Only use juices that have been freshly prepared by yourself using a juicer. Bought juices will not have the same therapeutic effect.

- A variation is to do a one-day mono-fruit fast using organic fruit. You could experiment with grapes (all colours and varieties), apples (all types), melons, mangos or papaya. A mono-fruit fast has a similar effect to a juice fast and is highly alkalising.

THE LIVER FLUSH

The following two liver flush regimes involve the juices of vegetables that are known to enhance liver function, and thus may be particularly helpful for people who are seeking to detoxify quite quickly. The combination of these juices, along with the olive oil, stimulates the liver to throw off accumulated toxins. Coffee is then taken as an enema, to encourage the liver to produce more bile, through which it eliminates waste products, thus helping the detoxification process (see later in this chapter). In some cases the sudden off-loading of toxins can make people feel unwell, just as often, however, people report a feeling of lightness, cleanliness and even euphoria.

One-day liver flush

1   At the beginning of the day it is recommended that you
     have a coffee enema (optional, see page 156).
2   Every hour, for eight hours, have a drink made from:
     ● 100 ml carrot juice
     ● 100 ml beetroot juice
     ● 100 ml filtered water
3   Three times during the day eat a salad made from:
     ● spinach
     ● carrots
     ● avocado
     ● courgettes
     ● a dressing made from olive oil and lemon juice
4   At the end of the day it is best to have a coffee enema or a
     colonic irrigation (see page 160). If you are unable to do
     this, have 2 teaspoons of psyllium husks dissolved in water,
     or in your juice if you find it more palatable.

Ten-day liver flush

1   Each day, on an empty stomach, have a drink made up of:
     ● the juice of 1 lemon
     ● 250 ml freshly made, organic carrot juice
     ● 3 tablespoons of extra-virgin olive oil
     ● a dash of cayenne pepper
2   Follow with a tea made from:
     ● fennel seeds
     ● fenugreek seeds
     ● lemon grass
     Use 2 teaspoons of each herb per 500 ml of filtered water,
     simmer gently, or steep in boiling water, for about 10

minutes. You can also add anise seeds, peppermint or a
few slices of ginger, to help take away the oily taste.

3 Do not eat for at least an hour afterwards.

4 Ideally have a coffee enema three times during the ten days
or a colonic irrigation at the end of the ten days. If this
is not possible, take 2 teaspoons of psyllium husks daily,
dissolved in either water or fresh juice.

THE GALL BLADDER FLUSH

The gall bladder flush might seem like quite an extreme
measure, but it can be very effective at encouraging a vigorous
emptying of the gall bladder, and can result in the removal of
smaller gallstones. It works because the oil stimulates the flow
of bile, while limonene, a component of lemons, is thought to
dissolve gallstones. It should not be done, however, if you have
largegallstones, as there is the possibility that they could get
stuck in the gall bladder duct, which would then necessitate
urgent surgery. For this reason it is important to have a correct
diagnosis from your doctor before attempting this flush.

I You need to prepare for the gall bladder flush five days in
advance by drinking at least three 225 ml glasses of freshly
made raw organic apple juice each day, in addition to meals.

2 On the morning of the sixth day, and on an empty stomach,
drink half a cup of extra-virgin olive oil mixed with the
juice of one lemon. Use a straw if you have difficulty
swallowing it. This should make you feel nauseous.

3 Lie on your right side for an hour, until you stop feeling
nauseous.

4 Do not eat for at least two hours after drinking the oil,
though frankly it is unlikely you will feel like doing so anyway.

5 To relieve any discomfort, such as nausea, headaches, bloating or pain on your right side, you can give yourself a coffee enema (see below).

6 On subsequent days, repeat steps 2–5 until you stop feeling nauseous altogether. This usually takes three to four days.

7 Drink plenty of freshly made carrot, lemon and beetroot juice during the flush, and for a week afterwards.

COFFEE AND CAMOMILE ENEMAS

Enemas involve injecting fluid (water, or water with other substances such as herbs) into the rectum and holding the fluid in for a period of time before expelling it. The water only reaches the lower portion of the colon. Although currently a fairly unfashionable therapy, they have been used since time immemorial as a means of cleansing. A translation of a 3rd-century Aramaic manuscript says, 'I tell you truly, the uncleanness within is greater by much than the uncleanness without. Renew your baptising with water [enemas] on every day of your fast, when you see that the water which flows out of you is as pure as the river's foam'. They remain popular on the Continent, where they are taken much more for granted than in the UK as a means of treatment.

Coffee enemas are particularly useful in helping the liver to detoxify, and give new meaning to the idea of taking a 'coffee break'. So give up your cup of coffee by all means, but don't throw away the packet! Coffee taken rectally goes to the liver via the portal vein and causes the bile duct to dilate. This is useful because it causes the release of bile already stored in the gall bladder, and so encourages the elimination of toxins into the bowels. Compounds in the palmitic acid found in coffee – kahweol and cafestol palmitate – promote the activity of glutathione-S-transferase, a major detoxification enzyme, when it reaches the liver via the portal vein. The effect of coffee enemas is likely to be quite limited, however, if done in isolation. They need to be carried out on a regular basis (say three times a week) or even better after a liver flush (described above) to be of any real use. Advocates suggest that because the coffee enema is retained for about 15 minutes, and because all the blood in the body passes through the liver once every three minutes, these enemas act as a form of dialysis of the blood.

Charlotte Gerson, daughter of Max Gerson who devised the Gerson Therapy (a serious detoxification programme for people who are very unwell), has lectured to medical students on the benefit of coffee enemas. She says, 'It is difficult to describe the incredulous facial expressions which ripple across a medical school lecture audience as the topic of coffee enemas is introduced . . .' A wise guy heckles, 'How do you take it?' 'Black – without cream and sugar!'

Coffee enemas were first used during the First World War and came about by accident. There was only enough morphine for use during operations and no painkillers for post-operative care. The surgeons, who were sometimes working 24–36 hours without a break, kept awake by drinking huge quantities of strong coffee. In the meantime, many of the soldiers were prescribed water enemas for their constipation, and the nurses, desperate for something to relieve their pain, reasoned that if the coffee was doing the doctors good, perhaps it would also help the patients. So leftover coffee from the pot was used for enemas, and the patients reported that they got pain relief from them.

There are several important pointers to remember if you are going to incorporate coffee enemas into your regime on a regular basis:

● If you have any bowel irritation, manifesting in conditions such as ulcerative colitis, Crohn's disease or diarrhoea you must not use coffee enemas. Instead use soothing and healing camomile enemas.

- If it turns out that you are hyper-sensitive to caffeine and get palpitations when doing the coffee enema, then this is a sign of toxicity. It should settle down if you continue with a detoxifying diet and the enemas after a few weeks. You may want to stop the enemas until you have followed a cleansing diet for a while first.

- Make sure that you drink enough fluid to avoid an electrolyte imbalance (electrolytes are minerals dissolved in solution – such as in our blood).

- Ideally, drink at least three freshly made juices for each coffee enema. This is to make sure that your liver is being supported and encouraged to eliminate toxins.

- If conducting regular coffee enemas it is important to follow a high nutrient diet that is rich in fruit and vegetables, to maintain mineral levels in the body.

- The enema does not travel up very far into the colon and the tube should only be inserted between 5 cm and an absolute maximum of 15 cm.

- Make sure that you are comfortable and warm while taking your enema. You have enough time to do some reading, to meditate or even to make a couple of phone calls!

- It is best to take the enema lying on your right side as there is better absorption into the haemorrhoidal veins on this side. The coffee is absorbed into the haemorrhoidal veins and is then taken into the portal system directly to the liver.

- Taking an enema for more than 15 minutes has little value, as experiments have shown that all the coffee is absorbed from the fluid by that time.

- The enema can cause the gall bladder to spasm and then

flush bile down the bile duct. The enema can also cause flatulence and gas as the bile goes through the intestinal tract. It is also possible for some bile to back up into the stomach and if this happens then lots of peppermint tea should be drunk to flush the bile out of the stomach.

- Use biodegradable, food-use detergent for keeping equipment clean and rinse with 6 per cent hydrogen peroxide.
- Be cautious about using coffee enemas without professional supervision if you have had large amounts of drugs previously, including chemotherapy. The enemas can cause sufficient off-loading of the drugs from the liver to cause a re-experiencing of the original toxic effects of the drugs.

To carry out a coffee enema, you need to buy an enema kit from your pharmacy, brew up some coffee as described below, resist the temptation to drink it, and follow the instructions that come with the kit. If you have not eaten, or are hungry, make sure that you eat a light meal first, perhaps of some fruit, as otherwise the enema may lead to a blood sugar low being experienced.

The enema is made by adding 3 tablespoons of organic ground coffee (not instant coffee) to 1 litre distilled water. (Do not use non-organic coffee as pesticides and other toxic material can be readily absorbed directly into the bloodstream.) Bring the water to the boil in a stainless steel, glass or enamel pot, add the coffee a little at a time to avoid boiling over, and boil for five minutes uncovered, to drive off the oils. Cover, lower the heat and simmer for 15 minutes. Strain through a fine mesh sieve and allow to cool to body temperature before using.

If you are making a camomile enema, use 50 g dried flowers and 1 litre distilled water. Bring the water to the boil, add the flowers and boil for five minutes. Turn down the heat and simmer for ten minutes. Strain, cool and use at body temperature.

If you wish, you can mix the coffee and camomile enemas together.

COLONIC IRRIGATION

Unlike enemas, colonic irrigation is not self-administered, and you need to find a reputable therapist. It is a procedure that does not appeal to everybody! Nevertheless, it has its uses in resolving long-term health problems, and can also be useful as part of a wider, long-term health programme to help resolve constipation, diarrhoea, digestive problems, low energy and laxative abuse.

The therapist inserts a tube into the rectum and, for 20 minutes or so, water is flushed up into the colon and drained out again. Unlike enemas, the water is flushed through the whole colon up to the junction with the small intestine. Depending on what is required of the therapy, the water that is injected is either at body temperature or cold – cold water is often used to tonify the muscular wall of the bowel. It is common to add some herbs to the final water flush to achieve a number of effects, such as speeding up detoxification of the liver. The active compounds in herbs are absorbed across the colon wall and have a therapeutic effect (in the same way that many medicines are administered by suppository, especially on the Continent).

A wide variety of health benefits are claimed for colonic irrigation, and it may seem as if these are too widely based. The main purpose of colonic irrigation is to clean the colon of a lifetime's accumulated debris. Faeces can accumulate in the folds of the colon, furring it up, causing auto-intoxication and a reduction in its effectiveness. It may seem incredible that this debris accumulates, but it can be compared to carbon waste accumulating, little by little, in a car exhaust, until it stops it working properly. Likewise, the encrusted faeces and mucus in some people's colons is sufficient to slow down the contractions of the colon, called peristalsis, needed for healthy elimination. Stress is also a major factor in slowing down peristalsis and the bowel is particularly sensitive to emotions such as repressed anger and grief. A combination of stress and long-term bad dietary habits is the cause of a lot of digestive and eliminative misery for many people. It is the improvement in the functioning of the body's detoxification channels, which are freed up by a newly effective colon, that leads to an improvement in general health.

It may take several treatments to achieve the desired effect, and it may then be recommended that further treatments are carried out at six- or 12-month intervals. Colonic irrigation is not appropriate for everyone and it is important to give the therapist a full breakdown of your health history in order that they can work out the best treatment plan. Colonics are not suitable for those with severe heart or cardiovascular disease, gastro-intestinal haemorrhage or perforation, severe haemorrhoids, colon cancer, bowel fissures, hernias, kidney disease or for those who are pregnant. It is an invasive procedure and I would always insist that the therapist uses disposable equipment. The procedure is not uncomfortable if correctly administered. If a number of colonics are being taken then it becomes quite important to 'reinoculate' the bowels with friendly bacteria. The process of flushing water throughout the colon can be fairly effective at partially removing unfriendly bacteria and candida (a yeast), however it is a good idea to replace the friendly bacteria which may have been washed out as well. This is simply done by adding a preparation of bacteria to the water in the final flush.

HERBAL COLON CLEANSING

If you feel that you would benefit from colon cleansing, but can't face the prospect of colonic irrigation, or if it is contra-indicated, you can use a herbal and fibre cleanse over a few months – it is slower, but just as effective, and is often a gentler option. There are many programmes and regimes available from different supplement companies, but in general they centre on mild herbals that encourage peristalsis and tonifying of the bowels, and fibres which bulk out the stools. Supplements and programmes usually also include psyllium, pumpkin seed husks and probiotic bacteria such as acidophilus.

I find that the simplest and most effective regime is to take one or two teaspoons daily of psyllium husks mixed in with juice. If you wish you can always use clay (see page 116). Use this regime over at least three months for a gentle colon cleanse. If you have bowel problems such as constipation start with ½ teaspoon of psyllium and build up to the full dose over two to four weeks.

CHAPTER ELEVEN

You Can Make a Difference

The 20th century saw a revolution in the way that humankind manipulated its environment. This skill of being able to alter our surroundings to suit our needs has been our strength as a species, and is what allowed us to migrate out of the savannas and survive no matter what the climate or conditions that surrounded us. But this skill may also lead to our downfall. At the beginning of the 21st century we are finally beginning to address the questions posed by this restructuring of our environment. What impact has our behaviour had on other species, on the plant life upon which we depend for producing oxygen, on the animals at the bottom of the food chain, and on our planet? What effect is our use of plastics, chemicals and high energy consumption having on our own health?

We are not all politically or environmentally motivated, and these questions may be too big, and too depressing for many people to want to think about. But even if your interest in the effects of pollution is motivated by the fact that you want to preserve and improve your health, you can console yourself with the knowledge that whatever you do to lead a more natural, and less toxic, life will also impact upon the health of the planet and therefore on the people, animals and plants around you. In a small way you will also be leaving a healthier legacy for the generations that follow.

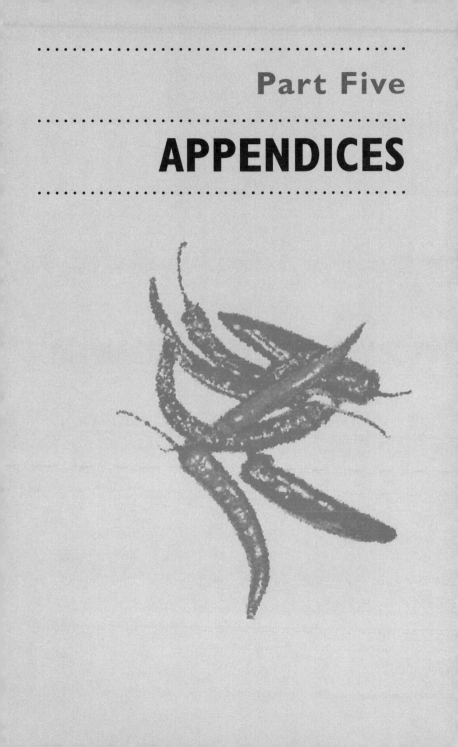

Part Five

APPENDICES

Cleansing Foods

Food/Herb	Liver support	Bile	Bowel	Kidney support	Blood cleansing/ lymph
FRUIT					
apples	★★		★		
apricots	★	★	★		
cranberries	★		★	★	
grapes (red)	★		★	★	★
guavas	★		★		
lemon	★	★			★
mangoes	★		★		
melon (yellow)	★		★		
papaya	★		★★		
pears	★		★★		
pineapple	★		★★		
plum (red)	★		★		★
pomegranate	★		★		
prunes	★		★★		
raspberries	★		★	★	★
watermelon	★		★		
VEGETABLES					
asparagus	★		★	★	★★
artichoke (globe)	★★★	★★	★		★
aubergines	★		★		★
avocado	★		★		

Food/Herb	Liver support	Bile	Bowel	Kidney support	Blood cleansing/ lymph
VEGETABLES					
beetroot	★★★		★		★
beans	★		★		
broccoli	★★★		★★		
Brussel sprouts	★★★		★★		
cabbage	★★★		★	★	
carrots	★★	★	★★	★	
cauliflower	★★★		★		
celery	★	★		★★	★★
cucumber	★		★	★	
fennel	★★		★	★★	★★
greens (dark, leafy)	★★★		★		★
kohlrabi	★★	★	★	★	
leeks	★★	★★	★★	★	
lettuce	★		★	★	★
olives	★				
onion	★★★		★		
parsnips	★		★	★	
peppers (bell)	★		★★		
pumpkin	★		★		
radishes	★★★		★	★	★
swede	★★★		★		
sweetcorn	★		★		
sweet potato	★		★	★	
tomatoes	★		★	★	★
turnip	★★★		★		
watercress	★★		★★		★

Food/Herb	Liver support	Bile	Bowel	Kidney support	Blood cleansing/ lymph
NUTS, SEEDS, BEANS					
almonds	★		★		
alphafa	★				
Brazil nuts	★★				
linseeds			★★		
pulses	★		★		
pumpkin seeds	★		★★	★	
sesame seeds	★		★		
soya beans	★	★			
sprouted pulses	★★		★		★
sprouted seeds	★★		★		
sunflower seeds	★		★		
tofu	★				
GRAINS					
brown/wild rice	★		★★★		
buckwheat	★		★★	★	
millet	★				★
sprouted barley juice	★★★			★★	★
sprouted wheat- grass juice	★★★			★★	★
MEAT AND EGGS					
eggs	★★	★			
liver (organic)	★	★			
oily fish	★	★			

Food/Herb	Liver support	Bile	Bowel	Kidney support	Blood cleansing/ lymph
HERBS AND SPICES					
aloe vera	★		★	★	★
burdock root	★			★	★
camomile flower	★				★
caraway			★		
cardamon			★		
cayenne pepper					★
cinnamon			★		
dandelion root	★★★	★	★★	★	★★
echinacea				★	★★★
garlic	★★		★	★	★★★
ginger					★
liquorice root	★		★★		
milk thistle	★★★				★
parsley			★★	★	★
peppermint		★★			
red clover					★★
rosemary	★★			★	★★
tarragon		★		★	
turmeric	★★★	★			★
vervain	★			★	
yellow dock	★				★★
MISC					
algae	★	★		★	★
green tea		★		★★	
lecithin	★★★		★★		
pine bark	★★				★★

Resources

To find out more about Suzannah Olivier's workshops, books and other activities see her website at: www.healthandnutrition.co.uk. Or email her at: eattobefit@aol.com

HERBAL AND NUTRIENT SUPPLEMENT SUPPLIERS

BIOCARE mail order: 0121 433 3727; also stocked by good independent health food shops
- nutrients: large range of vitamins, minerals and antioxidants
- liver support: HEP194, HepaGuard Forte, milk thistle
- liver and gall bladder: LIV243, beetroot extract
- kidneys: NEF242

BLACKMORES
Supply a full range of good herbs and nutrients for every need, available from good quality health food shops.

HEALTH PLUS Tel: 01323 492096
- nutrients: range of multi-nutrients supplied in convenient daily dose packs, each containing a combination of supplements designed for specific health conditions
- liver: Detox 2000, Detox pack (28-day supply)

HIGHER NATURE mail order: 01435 882880
- nutrients: range of vitamins, minerals and antioxidants

● detox: aloe detox, L-glutamine powder (nitrogen balance), MSM

LAMBERTS Tel: 01892 552120; available from good independent health food retailers
● nutrients: large range of vitamins, minerals and essential fats
● liver: Silymarin complex, L-methionine, L-glutathione.

LICHTWER PHARMA
Supply a range of herbal supplements, including Cynara Artichoke, available from large health food shops and chemists.

NUTRI LTD mail order: 0800 212742
● nutrients: a comprehensive range of vitamins, minerals and antioxidants
● liver: speciality detoxification formulas Ultra Clear and Ultra Clear Plus (which combine a number of ingredients, including N-acetyle cystein and L-glutamine), designed by leading nutritionist Jeffry Bland
They also stock tongue scrapers and a number of different fibre/colon cleanse programmes.

THE NUTRI CENTRE mail order: 020 7436 5122
Stock an extensive range of nutrition products, health foods and books from various suppliers and manufacturers. You can also visit their shop, which is in London, W1.

SOLGAR Tel: 01442 890355; stocked by good independent health food shops
● nutrients: a large range of low to high dose vitamins, minerals and antioxidants

- liver: milk thistle herb/seed, milk thistle and dandelion complex.

TO FIND A NUTRITIONAL THERAPIST

BRITISH ASSOCIATION OF NUTRITIONAL THERAPISTS (BANT) BCM BANT London WC1N 3XX Tel: 0870 6061284

For a list of registered nutrition therapists please send a large SAE to the above address.

INSTITUTE FOR OPTIMUM NUTRITION (ION) Blades Court, Deodar Road, London SW15 2NU. Tel: 020 8877 9993

BRITISH SOCIETY FOR ALLERGY ENVIRONMENTAL AND NUTRITIONAL MEDICINE (BSAENM) Tel: 01703 812 124 Website: www.bsaenm.org.uk

For a list of medical doctors who have a particular interest in nutritional medicine.

SOCIETY FOR THE PROMOTION OF NUTRITIONAL THERAPY PO Box 626, Woking GU22 0XD Tel: 01483 740 903

For information please send a SAE, plus £1, to the above address.

BREAKSPEAR HOSPITAL (private) Hemel Hempstead, Hertfordshire Tel: 01442 261333

They specialise in helping people with EI (environmental illness).

FOR COLONIC HEALTH

COLONICS INTERNATIONAL ASSOCIATION
16 Drumond Ride, Tring, Herts HP23 5DE Tel: 01442 827687
For a list of registered therapists send an SAE.

ROBERT GRAY INTESTINAL CLEANSING PROGRAM
Tel: 01342 410 303 for Best Care Products

BIOCHEMICAL TESTING

Most of these tests are only available through practitioners.
If you do obtain one that is available direct to the public,
you are strongly advised to have the results interpreted by
a nutritionist or other health professional so that the
appropriate action can be taken.

DIAGNOSTECH LTD Tel: 0800 731 5655
Liver detoxification capacity test

GREAT SMOKIES DIAGNOSTIC LABORATORY
The services of this laboratory, which offers liver detoxification
profiles and hair mineral analysis, can be obtained through
their two UK agents:
Diagnostic Services Ltd, tel: 0151 922 6200
Health Interlink Ltd, tel: 01582 794094

THE INDIVIDUAL WELLBEING DIAGNOSTIC
LABORATORY Tel: 020 7730 7010
Offer liver function tests, hair mineral analysis and allergy
tests. They run a clinic as well as a postal service. Tests are
supported by a nutrition consultation.

ORGANIC FOOD SOURCES

THE SOIL ASSOCIATION 86 Colston Street, Bristol, BS1 5BB
Tel: 0117 929 0661 website: www.soilassociation.org
Provide a list of organic suppliers in the UK, as well as
publications on organic issues. Telephone to check the
price of the catalogue.

SIMPLY ORGANIC nationwide 48-hour delivery Tel: 0845 1000
444 website: www.simplyorganic.net

WATER DISTILLER SUPPLIERS

WHOLISTIC RESEARCH COMPANY Tel: 01954 781074

HIGHER NATURE Tel: 01435 882880

AQUAPURE DISTILLATION Tel: 020 8892 9010

FRESHWATER FILTER COMPANY Tel: 020 8558 7495

THE FRESHWATER COMPANY Tel: 0345 023998
Delivery service, in the south east, of pre-distilled water.

SUPPLIERS OF JUICERS AND OTHER EQUIPMENT

WHOLISTIC RESEARCH COMPANY Tel: 01954 781074

THE FRESH NETWORK Tel: 0870 800 7070

SUPPLIERS OF ADDITIVE-FREE PERSONAL CARE AND HOUSEHOLD PRODUCTS

THE GREEN PEOPLE COMPANY LTD Tel: 01444 401444
   website: www.greenpeople.co.uk
In addition to personal care products, they also have an excellent herbal elixir with liver support herbs.

STEWART DISTRIBUTION Tel: 01273 625 988
Crystal Spring deodorant (aluminium, petroleum, perfume free).

NATURAL COLLECTION Tel: 01225 442288
   website: www.greenstore.co.uk

NATURAL WOMAN orderline: 0117 946 6649 (for a brochure)
Supply unbleached, natural cotton and women's hygiene products

NEAL'S YARD
Aromatherapy and natural products. Stocked at good quality stores. For your nearest stockist, call: 020 7498 1689

HEALTHY HOUSE Tel: 01453 752216

ELYSIA NATURAL SKIN CARE Tel: 01386 792 642

PITROCK LTD
Importers of tongue scrapers. You should find them at large health food shops and chemists, if not, consult their website at: www.pitrok.co.uk/tonguecleaner

BOOKS

The Sprouters Handbook Edward Cairney, Argyll Publishing (reprinted 1999)
The Healing Clay Michel Abehsera, Citadel Press (1994)

Recipe books

Raw Energy Recipes Leslie and Susannah Kenton, Ebury Press (1994)
The Optimum Health Cookbook Patrick Holford and Judith Ridgeway, Piatkus (1999)
Cooking Without Barbara Cousins, Thorsons (1998)
Gourmet Nutritional Therapy Cookbook Linda Lazarides, Waterfall (2000)

USEFUL WEBSITES

www.glutenfree-foods.co.uk
www.positivehealth.com
www.healthy.net
www.thinknatural.com
www.allergyfreedirect.co.uk
www.clearspring.co.uk

OTHER

National Radiological Protection Board (NRPB) Tel: 0800 614 529
For free infopack and information on radon levels in your area.

POCKET
BOOKS

NATURAL HORMONE BALANCE
YOU ARE WHAT YOU EAT
Suzannah Olivier

Women today are questioning the wisdom of
turning to artificial hormones and other chemical
preparations and techniques to alleviate their
female problems. A natural, nutritional approach
can help with PMS, infertility, mood swings,
irregular cycles, osteoporosis, endometriosis,
fibroids, ovarian cysts, breast cancer
and other problems.

Now all the nutritional advice you need is brought
together in **NATURAL HORMONE BALANCE**,
using simple, effective programmes that use
everyday foods and inexpensive diets.

Suzannah Olivier, a qualified nutritionist, has
written this major new health series fighting
common ailments the nutritional way.

ISBN 0 671 02954 1
Price £6.99

POCKET
B O O K S

BANISH BLOATING
YOU ARE WHAT YOU EAT
Suzannah Olivier

Many women, even if they are skinny, have a
problem with bloating and associated discomfort.

Now **BANISH BLOATING** looks at all the
possible causes – whether digestive, hormonal,
drug related or a sluggish detox process – and
pinpoints the best nutritional advice to combat this
condition. With easy-to-follow advice, and using
common, everyday foods and supplements, as
well as hit lists of food and food combinations to
avoid, here is the most healthy and holistic way to
eliminate the misery and discomfort of bloating.

Suzannah Olivier, a qualified nutritionist, has
written this major new health series fighting
common ailments the nutritional way.

ISBN 0 671 02953 3
Price £6.99

POCKET
BOOKS

MAXIMISING ENERGY
YOU ARE WHAT YOU EAT
Suzannah Olivier

We all want more energy.

MAXIMISING ENERGY shows how anyone, even
when juggling busy work and family lives, can
improve their available energy. Using tried and
trusted nutritional techniques, this book comes up
with a series of suggestions for maintaining a
steady stream of energy and good blood sugar
levels. It also highlights the foods and eating
habits that sap our bodies of energy.
MAXIMISING ENERGY will help eliminate
fatigue syndromes, listlessness and exhaustion on
a long-term basis.

Suzannah Olivier, a qualified nutritionist, has
written this major new health series fighting
common ailments the nutritional way.

ISBN 0 671 02955 X
Price £6.99

POCKET
BOOKS

EATING FOR A PERFECT PREGNANCY
YOU ARE WHAT YOU EAT
Suzannah Olivier

The pregnant mother's diet is of prime importance to the developing baby. Find out which are the best foods in **EATING FOR A PERFECT PREGNANCY**, a must-have book for expecting mothers. Covering pre-conception right through to breast feeding, this book advises on the impact that nutrition has on mother and child. Full of fascinating facts and practical advice, read this book for an energetic and symptom free pregnancy.

EATING FOR A PERFECT PREGNANCY continues the major new health series fighting common ailments the nutritional way. Suzannah Olivier, a qualified nutritionist, has written a groundbreaking series, which tailors detailed programmes to individual, common problems.

ISBN 0 671 03781 1
Price £6.99

POCKET
BOOKS

This book and other health and nutrition titles are available from
your bookshop or can be ordered direct from the publisher.

0 671 02954 1	**Natural Hormone Balance/Suzannah Olivier**	£6.99
0 671 02953 3	**Banish Bloating/Suzannah Olivier**	£6.99
0 671 02955 X	**Maximising Energy/Suzannah Olivier**	£6.99
0 671 03781 1	**Eating for a Perfect Pregnancy /Suzannah Olivier**	£6.99
0 671 77313 5	**Allergy Solutions/Suzannah Olivier**	£6.99
0 671 77377 1	**Potatoes Not Prozac/Kathleen DesMaisons**	£6.99
0 671 03735 8	**Food Your Miracle Medicine/Jean Carper**	£8.99
0 671 03736 6	**The Food Pharmacy/Jean Carper**	£8.99

Please send cheque or postal order for the value of the book, free
postage and packing within the UK; OVERSEAS including
Republic of Ireland £1 per book.

OR: Please debit this amount from my

VISA/ACCESS/MASTERCARD ....

CARD NO: ....

EXPIRY DATE ....

AMOUNT£ ....

NAME ....

ADDRESS ....

....

SIGNATURE ....

Send orders to SIMON & SCHUSTER CASH SALES
PO Box 29, Douglas Isle of Man, IM99 1BQ
Tel: 01624 836000, Fax: 01624 670923
www.bookpost.co.uk
Please allow 14 days for delivery. Prices and availability
subject to change without notice